Philosophy and Medicine

Founding Editors
H. Tristram Engelhardt Jr.
Stuart F. Spicker

Volume 149

Series Editors
Søren Holm, The University of Manchester, Manchester, UK
Lisa M. Rasmussen, UNC Charlotte, Charlotte, USA

Associate Editor
Jason Eberl, Health Care Ethics, Salus Ctr 501, Saint Louis Univ, Albert Gnaegi Center, St. Louis, MO, USA

Editorial Board Members
George Agich, Austin, USA
Bob Baker, Union College, Schenectady, USA
Jeffrey Bishop, Saint Louis University, St. Louis, USA
Ana Borovecki, University of Zagreb, Zagreb, Croatia
Ruiping Fan, City University of Hong Kong, Kowloon, Hong Kong
Volnei Garrafa, International Center for Bioethics and Humanities, University of Brasília, Brasília, Germany
D. Micah Hester, University of Arkansas for Medical Sciences, Little Rock, USA
Bjørn Hofmann, Norwegian University of Science and Technology, Gjøvik, Norway
Ana Iltis, Wake Forest University, Winston-Salem, USA
John Lantos, Childrens' Mercy, Kansas City, USA
Chris Tollefsen, University of South Carolina, Columbia, USA
Dr Teck Chuan Voo, Centre for Biomedical Ethics, Yong Loo Lin School of Medicine, National University of Singapore, Singapore, Singapore

The Philosophy and Medicine series is dedicated to publishing monographs and collections of essays that contribute importantly to scholarship in bioethics and the philosophy of medicine. The series addresses the full scope of issues in bioethics and philosophy of medicine, from euthanasia to justice and solidarity in health care, and from the concept of disease to the phenomenology of illness. The Philosophy and Medicine series places the scholarship of bioethics within studies of basic problems in the epistemology, ethics, and metaphysics of medicine. The series seeks to publish the best of philosophical work from around the world and from all philosophical traditions directed to health care and the biomedical sciences. Since its appearance in 1975, the series has created an intellectual and scholarly focal point that frames the field of the philosophy of medicine and bioethics. From its inception, the series has recognized the breadth of philosophical concerns made salient by the biomedical sciences and the health care professions. With over one hundred and twenty five volumes in print, no other series offers as substantial and significant a resource for philosophical scholarship regarding issues raised by medicine and the biomedical sciences.

Richard Sherlock

Medicine and Hope: A Natural Theology of Human Caretaking

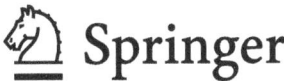 Springer

Richard Sherlock
Communication Studies and Philosophy
Utah State University
Logan, UT, USA

ISSN 0376-7418　　　　　　　ISSN 2215-0080　(electronic)
Philosophy and Medicine
ISBN 978-3-031-66484-7　　　ISBN 978-3-031-66485-4　(eBook)
https://doi.org/10.1007/978-3-031-66485-4

© The Editor(s) (if applicable) and The Author(s), under exclusive license to Springer Nature Switzerland AG 2024

This work is subject to copyright. All rights are solely and exclusively licensed by the Publisher, whether the whole or part of the material is concerned, specifically the rights of translation, reprinting, reuse of illustrations, recitation, broadcasting, reproduction on microfilms or in any other physical way, and transmission or information storage and retrieval, electronic adaptation, computer software, or by similar or dissimilar methodology now known or hereafter developed.

The use of general descriptive names, registered names, trademarks, service marks, etc. in this publication does not imply, even in the absence of a specific statement, that such names are exempt from the relevant protective laws and regulations and therefore free for general use.

The publisher, the authors and the editors are safe to assume that the advice and information in this book are believed to be true and accurate at the date of publication. Neither the publisher nor the authors or the editors give a warranty, expressed or implied, with respect to the material contained herein or for any errors or omissions that may have been made. The publisher remains neutral with regard to jurisdictional claims in published maps and institutional affiliations.

This Springer imprint is published by the registered company Springer Nature Switzerland AG
The registered company address is: Gewerbestrasse 11, 6330 Cham, Switzerland

If disposing of this product, please recycle the paper.

In memory of Arthur Dyck
Mentor Extraordinaire
In Corde Jesu

Preface

Aristotle, Aquinas, and many other thinkers have said that human beings are rational animals. This is obviously true. Whether human beings are the only rational animals has been heavily debated in recent years with the growth in serious thinking about the moral standing of animals; but it cannot be debated that reason is an essential aspect of human existence.

Hope is as much as reason an essential part of human life. Human beings rationally plan some future life or event. After they plan, however, they must hope that what they have planned for will come to pass. College students, for example, study for a satisfying and financially rewarding future. But they must hope that this future will come to pass. They cannot know that it will.

Persons hope for a better job, a good marriage, children, a better place to live, and thousands of other personal things they regard as good. Persons hope for peace on earth and prosperity for themselves and humanity in general. They hope for better earthly life and for many they hope for a life beyond bodily death.

What unites all of these hopes are two features: desire and uncertainty. We do not hope that the sun will rise in the east. It will. We do not hope that a plane traveling 800 miles an hour is breaking the sound barrier. It is. We do not hope that a pine tree will remain green all winter. It will.

When we hope we desire a good result that is uncertain. We make plans for something in the future that we regard as good, but this future is uncertain. Even religious people who claim to know that there is an eternal and blessed life after death with God must hope that they will be one of those who will be so blessed.

This book is about hope in one important part of human life: caretaking, especially medical caretaking. Hope is a crucial element in medicine. Patients hope that they can return to the life they had before they became ill. Doctors hope that they can successfully treat a patient's illness. Parents hope that their children's sickness can be successfully treated. Children hope that a parent's medical problem can be solved so that they can continue to have the mother and father that love them in the future.

The first chapter examines the concept of hope as it played a central role in thinking about medical ethics and practice in the last two centuries. We begin with the first important medical ethics work in modern times by Thomas Percival in 1803 in this work Percival says that doctors must be "ministers of hope" for their patients. Whether religious or not this has been a pervasive theme in thinking about medicine. Patients hope to recover their health. Doctors hope that their treatments will be successful.

The unfortunate part of this emphasis on hope has been the belief, until very recently, that to sustain hope for the patient and his family and his friends the patient must not be told the truth about his illness. In short, in order to sustain the patient's hope, he must be deceived or even lied to about his medical condition. This problem will also be treated in the first chapter.

There are two forms of uncertainty in medicine. The first form of uncertainty is when the doctor and the patient know what a good result should be from the doctor's treatment, e.g., have the patient able to walk around the block after a spinal fracture. But the physician is very uncertain whether he can achieve this result. The doctor has no doubt about what would be a good result. He and the patient must hope that this result can be achieved. I refer to this as noetic uncertainty.

The second form of uncertainty is when the doctor knows in a broad sense what is able to be achieved with this patient. What is uncertain is whether he or she should do it. For example, suppose a patient refuses a biopsy for possible cancer because of a patently false belief about air on a tumor causing it to spread. Should the doctor try to have him declared incompetent so that he can perform the biopsy anyway? I refer to this as moral uncertainty. In these cases, the uncertainty is not about whether the doctor is able to perform what is needed to be performed but whether the doctor should do it.

Chapters 2 and 3 consider these two forms of uncertainty and hope with actual and literary cases. Chapter 2 discusses noetic uncertainty and hope where the doctor knows what the result of his treatment should be but must hope that this result can be achieved.

Chapter 3 will treat what I have called moral uncertainty where the doctor knows what she can do but is uncertain whether this should be done. Suppose a patient who is otherwise fully rational and mentally stable refuses neurosurgery for a possible brain tumor with the simple statement "nobody is going to cut on my brain." Should the doctor try to have the patient declared incompetent so she can operate anyway?

Chapter 4 considers what I have called the "language of hope." In general hope requires desire and uncertainty. But many questions remain. Generally, persons desire what they believe to be a good result for themselves or others. Can it be hope when a person desires that another person suffers or has something horrible happened to them? Secondly how much uncertainty must there be. Must it only be unlikely or improbable? Can a doctor and patient hope for success when there is only a 10% chance of success? Can it be hope when fans hope that their team can win a championship when there is only a very small mathematical chance that they can do so? These issues will be discussed in this chapter.

There are two levels or forms of hope. The first form and most common is hope for an unexpected good in this world, e.g., an end to starvation, racism, and war. In medicine these hopes are pervasive: e.g., new forms of treatment for cancer, better treatment for those suffering from serious mental illness, new and more effective ways of delaying the progression of Alzheimer's. Temporal hopes are the subject of Chap. 5.

Beyond temporal hopes there are hopes for what I refer to as a transcendent good. Temporal hopes are for goods in this world based on what we know currently and how what we know may be extended to bring about a temporal good. Since we know a great deal about cancer we can hope for more effective and less painful treatments for cancer than chemotherapy. Given our expensive knowledge of the beginning of Alzheimer's we may hope for new and more successful ways of stopping or delaying the onset of Alzheimer's.

However, what if the doctor believes that during a complicated surgery the patient is almost certain to die? Family, friends, and even the doctor must hope that the patient will not die. The prediction that the patient will die is not a certainty. If the patient were dead, the doctor would not operate. Even in the most tragic and seemingly hopeless circumstances hope must require that the future remains open not closed. But this open future cannot be based on what we know about the world now. It must be based on a belief that we do not know all about reality. Something beyond or outside of what we know can bring about good out of what appears to be a lost cause where pain suffering and even death is all that can be expected. This sort of transcendent hope will be treated in my last chapter.

Cases

There are nine specific cases in this book; there are four each in Chaps. 2 and 3 and one in Chap. 6. These cases are an important part of my discussion of hope. They are detailed so that the reader can see how in specific medical situations help must play a central role. What they do is show in practice how help is essential in human caretaking in medicine. They represent a number of medical specialties: surgery, orthopedic surgery, neurology, psychiatry, oncology, urology, gastroenterology. This allows the reader to see how pervasive is the need for hope in medicine.

Logan, UT, USA   Richard Sherlock

Acknowledgments

My thinking about hope and medicine began years ago when I was a professor of moral theology at Fordham University. I was invited to give the keynote address at a meeting of the National Federation of Catholic Physician's Guilds. The genesis of this book was that address.

I taught medical ethics at the University of Tennessee Center for the Health Sciences for several years. As a result, most of the cases I have used in this book come from my personal experiences. They are properly revised with names changed for reasons of privacy.

Many friends have helped bring this book to press. Professor Christopher Tollefson brought this book proposal to the attention of my publisher, Springer. For this I am very grateful. Friends Harrison Kleiner, John Crosby, and Lyra Pitstick discussed the issues extensively with me and helped me clarify my thinking. Friends Susan McGinnis and Louise Griffiths Johnson help me make my argument clear to non-professionals. My son Thomas helped me put the manuscript in the form required by my publisher. Finally, my editor Nagarnijan Paramasivam has helped my work in ways too numerous to mention.

All remaining mistakes and uncertainties are my responsibility alone.

Contents

1	**Hope and Medicine**	1
	I	2
	II	4
	III.	4
	IV	6
	V	13
	VI	16
2	**Epistemic Uncertainty**	19
	I Can the Doctor Achieve what he Knows is Right	19
	II Cases	20
	Charles (Chuck)	20
	Margaret Dolan	21
	Claire Darlington	23
	Dan Kelly	24
	III The Plague	26
	IV Examinig the Cases	29
	V	32
3	**Moral Uncertainty in Medicine**	35
	I Cases	35
	Vicki Cline	36
	Mark Willis	37
	Ken Tidwell	39
	Linda Janko	40
	II Equus	41
	III Examing the Cases	44
	IV	47

4	The Language of Hope	49
	I	50
	II	50
	III	51
	Hope and Uncertainty	51
	IV	54
	Hope and the Good	54
	V	57
	Conclusion	58
5	Hope and Temporal Goods	61
	I Socialism and Temporal Hope	62
	II	63
	III	65
6	Hope and Transcendence	75
	I Gabriel Marcel: Hope and Transcendence	76
	II Problem and Mystery	77
	III Faith	82
	IV Hope	85
	V Belif, Faith and Hope	90

Cases	93
Bibliography	95
Author Index	101
Subject Index	103

Chapter 1
Hope and Medicine

In 1803 63-year-old Scottish physician Thomas Percival published the first important modern work in medical ethics: *Medical Ethics or a Code of Institutes and Precepts Adapted to the Professional Conduct of Physicians and Surgeons*. The long part of the title was a commonplace of the time. It offered what amounted to a short abstract of the book. For over a century Percival's *Medical Ethics* was the dominant work of its kind in the English-speaking world. The first code of ethics of the newly formed American Medical Association, in 1849, was mostly taken word for word from Percival. While not as "word for word" from Percival, the first revision of the AMA code, in 1903, was almost wholly based on Percival's work.[1]

Much of Percival's prescriptions are still sound today, over 200 years later. The emphasis on confidentiality and "secrecy", the respect due physicians, the care they must devote to seeing patients, are still important.[2] So too is the emphasis on attending to patient needs without considering whether they can pay for their care. Though this last moral prescription is not followed as well as Percival might have liked[3] There is also a good deal of what we might call "medical etiquette" in Percival's work as well as a stress on the virtuous character and moral probity required for physicians.

---

[1] Thomas Percival, *Medical Ethics or a Code of institutes and Precepts Adapted to the Professional Interests of Physicians and Surgeons* (Manchester: S Russel, 1803) reprint (Leopold Classic Library, 2016) Also reprinted *Percival's Medical Ethics* ed. Chauncey Leake (Baltimore: Williams and Wilkins, 1927). For further reading: Ivan Waddington, "The Development of Medical Ethics" *Medical History* 19(1975): 38–51; Lisbeth Haakansson, *Medicine and Morals in The Enlightenment* (Amsterdam: Rodophi, 1997).
[2] Percival (1927), p. 90.
[3] Ibid. p. 99.

I

Three points discussed by Percival are today: (1) ignored, (2) given a completely different interpretation, or (3) rejected by writers on medical ethics, whether physicians, philosophers, or moral theologians and by the moral codes of professional societies.

Two of these points are deeply connected. They are also fundamentally ignored by medical societies, groups, and individuals who want medicine to be only a science, and to not be at all connected to what we might broadly call religion or faith. However, medicine and faith have always gone together. It is only in the last century that medical practice has tried to separate the two, to the detriment of both religion and medical practice. The third point that Percival makes is quite property rejected. This point will be treated later in this chapter.

Percival writes about the first two points thus:

> The physician should be a minister of hope and comfort to the sick that by such cordials to the drooping spirit he may smooth the bed of death, revive expiring life, and counteract the depressing of those maladies which rob the philosopher of fortitude and the Christian of consolation.[4]

Two interconnected ideas are found in this passage. The first is the idea that the physician is a sort of "minister" to the patient. The second is that the physician must treat the patient with hope for the patient's future, whatever that future may be.

As befits a Scottish Calvinist of the eighteenth century Percival's work has many explicitly Christian themes and references. Physicians should attend church regularly. They should not attend to patients on Sunday unless absolutely necessary. As he writes "The observance of the sabbath is a duty to which medical men are bound so far as is compatible with the urgency of the cases under their charge".[5]

In brief, Percival appears to hold that the physician should be a devout Christian, who carefully attends to Christian rituals and lives a life of Christian character. When he says "minister" he envisions someone like a Christian clergyman. The physician "ministers" to the needs of the body. While the clergyman ministers to the needs of the soul.

Even in Percival, however, this supposedly neat division of patient needs, and professional responsibilities breaks down. The breakdown is evident precisely in this quote we are examining. The physician (not just the clergyman) should be a "minister of hope". In another passage he writes that "Humanity and the welfare of the sick man commonly require that his drooping spirit be revived by every encouragement and hope which can honestly be suggested to him" Percival does not council outright "lies" to the patient. But the "whole truth" need not be conveyed, lest

---

[4] Ibid. p. 91.
[5] Ibid. p. 108.

this will depress the patient. "The physician is at liberty to say little. But let that little be true".[6]

The rest of this work is one modest attempt to develop the central insight of Percival's claim. The importance of hope in human caretaking and the physician who grounds his caretaking both in science and hope for and with the patient. This hope is ultimately that good will triumph over that which is not good i.e., bad, or evil.

All human caretaking, in my view, seeks the good of those for whom one cares. Wives and husbands care for the good of each other. Parents care for the good of their children. Counselors care for the good of those whom they counsel. Medical professionals care for the good of their patients. In almost all instances this caring for the other is not based on certainty about the good being realized for those who are cared for. It is based on hope. As we shall see later, hope is not certainty. A person hopes for what is desirable but uncertain.

There are, I believe, two types of uncertainty in medicine which will be examined in separate later chapters. The first is what I call noetic or epistemic uncertainty. This is where the professional knows what the right thing to do or refrain from doing is, but is uncertain whether she can achieve this goal, whether she can successfully treat the patient, or if for good reasons she refuses to do what the patient desires, she must hope that worse results will not follow. The physician knows what the right thing to do or not do is. But the physician must hope that good results will follow.

The second type of uncertainty is what I call moral uncertainty. In these cases, the physician is relatively certain what he can do or not do but is very uncertain about whether the result of his action will bring about good for the patient.

In what follows in this chapter we shall examine how Percival's work deeply influenced writings in medical ethics and the codes of medical ethics in the rest of the nineteenth century and well into the twentieth. Further, we shall see how the emphasis on hope has influenced medical thinking and practice even in the last few decades.

After this review I shall carefully examine the two forms of uncertainty and hope we have just noted with practical cases and important thinkers. There is a separate chapter on the language of hope. Then we will examine two sorts of hope. First will be temporal hopes for temporal goods, e.g., a better job, more income, a spouse, physical health. Second will be transcendent hopes for a transcendent good, possibly from a transcendent source e.g., what many would call a miracle or an afterlife.

---

[6] Ibid. pp. 187–188.

II

There are two bodies of literature related to hope that I will not engage in this discussion. The first is the vast body psychological material about hope and optimism and the importance of hopefulness in mental health. I have read a good deal of this material, but I am not an expert in this field, and I am not competent assess or employ it in this discussion.[7]

The second body of material comes explicitly from theology, primarily protestant theology. In the 1960s and into the 1970s there was a great deal of discussion about the "theology of hope" spurred on by an important book by that name from a well-known and influential German reformed theologian Jurgen Moltmann. This discussion also engaged other well-known protestant thinkers, e.g. the Lutherans Carl Brataan, and Wolfhart Pannenberg Congregationalist Fredrick Herzog, and Brazilian presbyterian Rubem Alves. Also involved was the important Catholic theologian, Karl Rahner. This large body of literature focuses on understanding Christianity as a religion of eschatological hope. The message of this literature is an eschatological future in which God brings about a divinely grounded good.[8]

This literature is interesting, but it is only tangentially relevant here. Some of it will be referenced in the chapter on earthly, temporal hopes, because the Marxist thinker we discuss there, Ernst Bloch and his massive work, *The Principle of Hope*, was highly influential in the origin of Moltmann's early work. Though I have studied this work closely, it does not deal with the sorts of personal caretaking issues I am treating in this volume.

III

We shall return to Percival's discussion of truth in medicine later. For now, let us think about the second word in the phrase "minister of hope" i.e., hope. The concept of hope is much under analyzed in both theology and philosophy. Consider the three "theological virtues" of medieval Christian thought, i.e., faith, hope and love.

---

[7] For an excellent overview and analysis: Adrienne Martin, *How we Hope: A Moral Psychology*. (Princeton: Princeton University Press, 2016); Also Elizabeth Hopper, "The Psychology of Hope" *Health Psychology* July, 6, 2020. Health Psychology; G. Alarcon et al. "Great Expectations: A Meta-Analytic Examination of Optimism and Hope", *Personality and Individual Differences* 54(2013): 821–827.

[8] Jurgen Moltmann, *Theology of Hope; On the Ground and Implications of Christian Eschatology.* trans. James Leitch (London: SCM Press, 1967); Carl Braatan, *The Future of God: The Revolutionary Dynamics of Hope*. (New York,: Harper and Row, 1969); Wolfhart Pannenberg, *Theology and the Kingdom of God* ed Richard John Neuhaus. (Philadelphia: Westminster Press, 1969); Fredrick Herzog, *A Theology of Liberation*. (New York: Seabury Press, 1972); Rubem Alves, *A Theology of Human Hope*. (Washington D.C.: Corpus Books, 1971). Also see Douglas Meeks, *Origins of the Theology of Hope*. (Philadelphia: Fortress Press, 1974); Jessica Murdoch, "Between Heaven and History: Rahner on Hope." *New Blackfriars*. 95(2014): 263–284.

An enormous amount has been written about "love" or what is often called "charity". What is Christian love's relation to social justice or political regimes? How is it related to other forms of human relationships analyzed in the classical world: Eros (Plato's *Symposium*) and Philia (friendship) books 8 and 9 of Aristotle's *Nichomachean Ethics* or Plato's *Lysis*. Unfortunately, in modernity we have largely reduced eros to the sexually "erotic."[9]

The same is true of faith. A substantial amount exists about faith. What is faith, especially religious faith? What is the relation between faith and belief? Between faith and knowledge? Is faith a gift from God? What is the relation between faith in God and rational arguments for the existence of God such as those given by Aquinas or Anselm?[10]

Hope, however, is much less studied. There is some philosophical work on hope but much of it is not very helpful. There is some theological work on hope but much of it, is too explicitly theological to be of real help in using the idea of hope in the interdisciplinary manner that Percival's use of the concept requires. We shall return to a discussion of some of this material, especially Aquinas' analysis of the virtue of hope.

As will be seen in subsequent chapters, the concept of hope is complex. For now, we can say, broadly, that hope takes over when certainty or high probability are no longer appropriate in the given situation. If I drop a rock from 5 feet above the ground, I do not hope it will hit the ground. I do not hope that the sun will arise in the east in the morning. If I mix two chemicals together, I do not hope for a certain result. In these cases, and thousands of others, I know, that the sun will come up in the morning, that the rock will drop down and there will be a specific result in a chemistry experiment.

So also hope seems out of place where a result seems highly probable. When a trained meteorologist predicts with 90% reliability that there will be snow during the morning commute, it seems not quite right to say that a skier "hopes" for snow. When a professor has announced that there will be an exam on the third Thursday of the semester it would be odd to hope that there will not be an exam.

---

[9] A few titles with references to more: Adrienne Moore ed. *The Routledge Handbook of Love in Philosophy.* (New York: Routledge, 2018); L. Blum, *Friendship, Altruism and Morality.* (New York: Routledge, 1980); R. Brown, *Analyzing Love.* (London: Cambridge, 1987); B. Helm, *Love, Friendship, and the Self.* (London: Oxford, 2010); I Singer. *The Nature of Love*. 3 vols. (Chicago: University of Chicago Press, 1984–1989); A Soble ed. *Eros, Agape, and Friendship: Readings in the Philosophy of Love.* (New York: Paragon, 1989); Dietrich von Hildebrand *The Nature of Love* trans. John Crosby, (Notre Dame: St. Augustine, 2010); C.S Lewis, *The Four Loves.* (New York: Harper, 2017).

[10] A few titles with references to more. John Hick, *Faith and Knowledge.* (Ithaca: Cornell University Press, 1966); Paul Helm, *Faith with Reason.* (London: Oxford University Press, 2000); Laura Callahan and Timothy O'Connor eds. *Religious Faith and Intellectual Virtue.* (London: Oxford University Press, 2014); Anthony Kenney. *What is Faith?* (London: Oxford University Press, 1992); William Sessions, *The Concept of Faith.* (Ithaca: Cornell University Press, 1994); Terence Penelhum ed. *Faith* (London: Collier Macmillan, 1989); T.C. O'Brien, *Faith in St. Thomas Aquinas*. (London: Blackfriars, 1974).

Of course, in both of these cases one is less certain than in the cases of the sun and the rock. It might not snow. It might rain instead. The professor might get sick. There might be a fire or a campus tragedy.

When certainty or high probability seem too strong then hope rightly captures our emotions and our reasons. When the sky is overcast, I can hope that at noon the sun will come out. When a baseball team is 10 games behind with 15 left to play, I can hope that they can win the championship. When I have not done very well on practice tests, I can hope that on the actual LSAT (Law School Admission Test) I can do well enough to be admitted to a good law school.

IV

The first code of ethics of the newly formed American Medical Association, adopted in 1849, employs, almost word for word, much of Percival's work, a fact which they willingly admit. "The committee which prepared this code …have carefully preserved the words of Percival whenever they preserved the precepts it wished to inculcate".[11]

Like Percival, the AMA in the nineteenth century directly connected medical ethics to religion. The opening line of the introduction reads: "Medical ethics, as a branch of general ethics must rest on the basis religion and morality". The preface also views physicians as agents of "providence", i.e., divine providence.[12]

Following Percival, this code also stresses that physicians should be persons of "high moral character." In attending to a patient with a fatal illness physicians have "a moral duty which is independent of and far superior to all pecuniary considerations." Furthermore, physicians should "evince a genuine love of virtue". Many other passages could be cited where the code speaks of the necessary moral probity and virtuous character of the physician.[13]

With respect to the topic, we have analyzed from Percival, the AMA takes his view directly with some additions. "The physician should the minister of hope and comfort to the sick, that by such cordials to the drooping spirit, he may smooth the bed of death, revive expiring life, and counteract the depressing influence of those maladies which often disturb the tranquility of the most resigned in their last moments"[14] Furthermore, the AMA noted something that was often lost sight of in medicine for the next century i.e. the importance of "bedside manner": "The life of a sick person can be shortened not only by the acts but also by the words or manner

---

[11] For a reprint: Arthur Dyck, William Curran, Stanley Reiser eds. *Ethics in Medicine: Historical Perspectives and Contemporary Concerns*. (Cambridge: MIT Press, 1977) pp. 26–33.

[12] AMA Code p. 26.

[13] To quote the code: "There is no profession from the members of which greater purity of character and a higher standard of moral excellence are required than the medical; and to attain such eminence is a duty every physician owes alike to his profession and to his patients" op. cit. p. 31.

[14] Ibid. p. 29.

of a physician. It is therefore a sacred duty to guard himself carefully in this respect and to avoid that which may have a tendency to discourage the patient and depress his spirits".[15]

Though not informing the patient of his or her serious situation was required, the physician "should not fail on proper occasions to give to the friends of the patient timely notice of danger." What Percival and the physicians of the nineteenth century should have known from experience is that their advice to inform the friends and family of the patient, but not the patient makes worse the hopeless feeling of the patient that they are trying to avoid. Patients can see in the faces of friends, in the eyes and voice of family that that something dreadfully wrong is known by everybody else, but not by them. The physician may be able to control his voice and demeanor. But those closer to the patient and less experienced in such control rarely can. On this point the data and clinical experience is clear. The worst situation for the patient is when bad news seems to be known by everybody else, and the patient does not.[16]

This practice was rooted in the belief that since the hope of the patient that he or she will get well is essential to the patient actually getting well, this hope should be supported by the physician. The physician (and other caretakers) should frequently tell the patient that they will recover when the physician believes otherwise. Or, at a minimum, the physician should do nothing to discourage the patients belief that they will get well. The patient had no right to the truth, if the physician did not believe that it would benefit the patient.

This position of Percival and the early AMA was reflected in a number of writers and physicians in the nineteenth and into the twentieth century.[17] One memorable example is from Oliver Wendell Holmes sr., friend of Emerson, Thoreau and other "transcendentalists", and father of the supreme court justice Oliver Wendell Holmes jr. Holmes sr. was then professor of medicine at Harvard. In a speech to the graduating class of the Bellevue Hospital College in 1871 he put the point directly: "The patient has no more right to all the truth you know than he has to all the medicine you carry with you in your saddlebags." The reason Holmes gives is right out of Percival's playbook: "It is a terrible thing to take away hope, even earthly hope, from a fellow creature."

He further advised the new physicians to create an important sounding name for a fictitious illness that can satisfy the patient who really desires to know what illness they have. If the physician appears to know the illness of the patient, then the patient can really trust that physician can bring them back to health. He advised them not to

---

[15] Idem.

[16] p. 30.

[17] John Gregory, *Duties and Qualifications of a Physician*. (London: Strahan and Cadell, 1772); Jules Styap, *A Code of Medical Ethics*. (London: Churchill, 1870); Andrew Wear and Johanna Kordesch eds. *Doctors and Ethics: The Earlier Setting of Professional Ethics*. (Amsterdam: Rodophi, 1993); Robert Baker, Dorothy Porter, Roger Porter eds. *The Codification of Medical Morality: Historical and Philosophical Studies in the Formalization of Western Medical Morality*. (New York: Springer, 1992).

use the name of an actual disease because some patients might actually look up that disease in books. Better to have a name that sounds important but which they will never find described in any book. Holmes told the graduating class that his personal favorite serious sounding, but fictitious name was "congestion of the portal system".[18]

This advice from Holmes is rooted in the same twin convictions of Percival. First is the belief that hope is essential for the patient getting well. In short, the patient's hope that he will recover is crucial for his really getting well. The second conviction was that to sustain the hope of the patient he or she must not be told the truth of how serious their condition is. This sort of truth will only depress patients and cause them to lose the hope necessary for their getting well.

A revised AMA code was adopted at the 1903 convention of the American Medical Association in New Orleans. This revised code is less wordy and somewhat more general than its predecessor. It is also deliberately not referred to as a "code of medical ethics". Rather it is titled a "principle of medical ethics". This is because the AMA wanted to leave as much freedom as possible for state and local medical associations to develop more specific codes. "Large discretionary powers are thus left to the respective state and territorial societies to form such codes and establish such rules for the professional conduct of their members as they may consider proper".[19]

This set of "principles" is not as openly religious as was the first "code". It does not say that practical ethics is a branch of "religion and morality" Whatever is meant by these broad and vague terms. In 1849 "religion" almost certainly meant protestant Christianity. Morality undoubtedly meant the common morality of ordinary persons, not the technical work of Aristotle, Aquinas, Bentham, or Kant.

On the central question of our study, however, the 1903 "principles" mirrors the position of Percival, the 1849 code, and Holmes. "The physician should not be forward to make gloomy prognostications". Such announcements will, of course, depress the patient and cause him or her to lose that hope that is crucial to regaining their health. However, as Percival and the AMA noted before, the physician should tell the truth to the family and friends of the patient.

Just as Percival, Holmes, and the previous code this revision states directly: "the physician should be a minister of hope and comfort to the sick" Furthermore, "the life of the patient may be lengthened or shortened not only by what the physician does or doesn't do but by what the physician says". According to the AMA at the turn of the twentieth century, the physician has a "solemn duty to avoid all utterances and actions having a tendency to discourage and depress the patient" In another way of stating it, do not do or say anything that might undermine the hope of the patient that he or she will get well.[20]

---

[18] Oliver Wendell Holmes, "The Young Practitioner" in *Medical Essays! 842–1882*. (Boston: 1891) p. 164–165. Retrieved from Project Guttenberg.

[19] *Revised AMA Code* (Cleveland Press, 1903).

[20] Ibid. sect. 6.

The AMA here does not specifically advise lying to the patient, as Holmes does. But they do say that in almost all situations truth that might depress the patient should not be given. Judicious council that will promote and strengthen "the good resolutions of the patient" if "tactfully offered" are helpful. But avoid anything that will undermine optimism and hope in the patient. Unlike more current codes for physicians, these "principles" like the earlier code also stresses the needed moral character of the physician: "there is no profession from the members of which greater purity of character and a higher standard of moral excellence are required than the medical" Though medical ethics writers today mostly ignore this requirement, something can be said for this point. How can a patient trust a physician to care for them, when the physician has not taken care of himself very well?

The tradition of Percival, Holmes and the early American Medical Association carried on well into the twentieth century. Doctors must sustain the hope of the patient, by lying or just not telling the truth if necessary.

In a famous essay in *Harper's Monthly* in 1927, physician Joseph Collins makes this point powerfully. He states bluntly that: "In forty years of contact with the sick" the patients who "couragesly want to know the truth could be counted on the fingers of one hand".[21]

Collins believes that while many patients say they want to know the truth almost all only want good news. They do not want to know the truth that they have a serious, possibly fatal illness. In his defense he offers examples of patients who, he believes, were benefitted by not being told the truth. For example, a patient who, "if he had been told that he had a disease which was universally believed to be progressive, apprehension would have depressed him so heavily that he would not have been able to offer resistance to its encroachment" Lying sustained his hope which was essential to his becoming well. In another example, he presents the case of a business executive, who, being told the truth about his condition and the prognosis, became so depressed that he committed suicide.

As Percival and Holmes, Collins holds that patients claim to want to know the truth. But almost all of them really do not. They do not want to know. Furthermore, knowing a harsh truth will harm them by causing them to lose hope of a future life of happiness. "The longer I practice medicine, the more I am convinced that every physician cultivate the fine art of lying".[22]

Collins notes that some lies told by physicians are for their own benefit. These may be told so that the physician can avoid a difficult conversation with the patient. Such deceptions as these are always wrong. There are other lies, however, which "contribute enormously to the physician's mission of mercy and salvation" Collins makes a clear distinction between doctors lying for their benefit and lying for the benefit of the patient, to help prevent the patient from becoming severely

---

[21] Joseph Collins "Should Doctors Tell the Truth." *Harpers Monthly Magazine*. 155 (1927): 320–326.
[22] Ibid. p. 321.

depressed and losing hope. The former the physician must never do. The latter he morally must do.

Another example of the power of the Percival tradition in both its positive and questionable elements is from 20 years after Collins, this time in a medical journal. The title is direct "Should the Cancer Victim be Told the Truth?" The answer is equally direct, NO. The patient should not be told that his disease is cancer "except in those uncommon instances in which special circumstances are present".[23]

Later, in the same essay, he writes of the "tension in medicine between the desire to follow the general moral rule of honesty in human relations and what he sees as the need in medicine not always to do so".

"Throughout my life I have been quite busy trying to align my conduct with principles inscribed on the tablets handed to Moses on Sinai, with the Sermon on the Mount and the Golden Rule in particular and with the formal ethical code governing the practice of medicine" On the tension between the general rule of honesty and what he sees as the needs of medical practice, the formal codes were silent.[24]

In a powerful statement he continued:

> I went even further afield in the attempt to square conscience with desire. I sought for the judgment of other men whose opinions command respect and I found them. Old Oliver Wendell Holmes concedes that "truth is for other worlds, hope is for this", Voltaire helps out with, "there are truths that are not for all men, nor for all time", Emerson, the beloved sage of Concord, says God gives to every mind the choice between truth and repose, take what you please, you can never have both. ... Even that arch cynic Anatole France said 'love the truth I believe humanity has need of it. But assuredly it has much greater need still of the untruth which consoles it and gives it infinite hope.[25]

A number of other physicians of the same time can be cited who still held to the Percival tradition in both in problematic and positive principles. Sustain the hope of the patient by not telling him or her harsh truths. In a 1953 study of Philadelphia physicians over two thirds of these practitioners did not tell patients about a diagnosis of cancer. Of the physicians in this study who specifically cared for patients with cancer three fourths almost never told patients the truth.[26]

The most well-known and well-designed of these studies was published in the *Journal of the American Medical* Association in 1961. This was a study of 219 physicians in a hospital in Chicago. The specialties represented were ob-gyn, surgery, oncology, neurosurgery, thoracic surgery, and orthopedics. The researcher, Donald Oaken, wanted to know what the policy of these physicians was about telling cancer patients the truth about their situation. He also wanted to know the source of

---

[23] M.G. Selig, "Should the Cancer Victim be told the truth" *Journal of the Missouri Medical Association.* 40(1943):33–35.

[24] Ibid. p. 34.

[25] Idem.

[26] Charles Wood, "The Doctor, The Patient, and The Truth" *Annals of Internal Medicine.* 24(1946): pp. 955–959; William Fitts and I.S. Bowden "What Philadelphia Physicians Tell Cancer Patients" *JAMA* 153 (1953): 901–904.

their policy. Was it what they were taught? Was it personal experience? Was it other emotional factors? Dr. Oaken received an astounding 95% response rate.[27]

What was the result? "There is a strong and general tendency to withhold this information". Almost 90% is within this half of the scale. Indeed, a majority tell only very rarely "What do these physicians tell patients if not the truth?" Euphemisms are the general rule. Mass, lesion, growth, benign tumor. "Some physicians avoid even the slightest suggestion of neo-plasia and quite specifically substitute another diagnosis"[28]

The reason these physicians do not tell the truth is right out of Percival's playbook. "Variations in approach also converge on a single major goal, the maintenance of hope. No inference was necessary to elicit this finding. Every single physician interviewed spontaneously emphasized this point and indicated his resolute and determined purpose is to sustain and bolster the patient's hope".[29]

Where did these physicians get this conviction that deception was necessary to sustain hope. Overwhelmingly they got this conviction from clinical experience. They seemed not to learn it from their training or from writings such as Percival, Holmes, or Collins. It was their experience that was the basis of their adopting the tradition of these previous writers.

Even later in the 1960s there is a powerful example of the persistence of the Percival tradition in both of its parts, as well as a rich example of the flaws in the insistence of this tradition in not telling the patient the truth about his or her condition In 1965 a young, Swiss trained psychiatrist at the University of Chicago was approached by a group of students from the Chicago Theological Seminary. Her name was Elizabeth Kubler-Ross. She would become world famous but at the time she was only a junior faculty member and clinician.[30]

These theological students would become pastors of churches and counselors to those undergoing the stresses and traumas of human life. They wanted to talk to persons in the hospital who were terminally ill. After all pastors, priests, and rabbis are often the first persons, after family, that are called when someone finds out that they are terminally ill. These students were planning careers as leaders of protestant churches. They obviously, and correctly, thought it would be helpful to have some experience with dying persons before they were ordained to be pastors of churches and counselors to those who were dying and their families.

The plan was that Dr. Kubler-Ross, the professional, would do the actual interview and the students would watch and take notes. After the interview or several interviews, the students and Dr. Kubler-Ross would have a seminar about what they learned, from the patient. The students and Dr. Kubler-Ross did not just want to read about death or statistical studies about those who are dying and their families and

---

[27] Donald Oaken, "What to tell Cancer Patients" *JAMA* 175(1961): 1120–1128. Reprinted in Dyck, Curran and Reiser eds. op. cit. pp. 224–235.
[28] Ibid.
[29] Ibid.
[30] Elizabeth Kubler-Ross *On Death and Dying*. (New York: Macmillan, 1969) pp. 1–20.

friends. They wanted to learn from those who were terminally ill themselves, who they regarded as the best teachers. The students and Dr. Kubler-Ross had the plan all set[31]

Kubler-Ross set about trying to locate such patients in the hospital. Surely there must be several. Talking to colleagues in surgery, gynecology, and internal medicine she could not find one doctor who would allow her and the students to interview such a patient. In their defense, she admits that she was new at the hospital and her colleagues did not know her well. Mostly, however, the physicians thought their patients were too weak, too tired, or too fragile to talk about their situation. In effect, they would lose hope if confronted with the truth. To quote her account: "a nurse angrily asked in utter disbelief if I enjoyed telling a twenty-year-old man that he had only a few weeks to live. She walked away before I could tell her more about our plans"[32]

However, contrary to the physicians who held on to the tradition of Percival, Holmes, and the early AMA, when Kubler-Ross and the students were actually able to talk to patients who were terminally ill they were "welcomed with open arms." The persons who were in these traumatic situations wanted to talk. What sustained them in their last weeks and months was hope, i.e., the best part of the Percival tradition. Contrary to the tradition we have examined hope and honesty, or openness were not opposed to each other. They were most often allies of sorts. These persons kept their hope alive even in the most difficult circumstances. "The most realistic patients" left the possibility open for a cure: "a new drug, a new surgery, a new research project".[33]

Yet this hope that sustains these persons "through days, weeks, months of suffering "is rooted more deeply than the hope for a cure" or what we might call a "miracle". It is a belief or "feeling that all of this must have some meaning." This hope for the triumph of some good, over what they and the persons around them, both professionals and family, regard as evil or horrible sustains them in the most trying circumstances. "It gives the terminally ill a sense of a special mission in life which helps them maintain their spirits," through more tests, procedures, and suffering.

These patients had great faith in their doctors and other professionals who cared for them. They had great confidence in the doctors who shared this hope with them. When "we share this hope with them" the patients have a better life, no matter how short their future may be. Physicians should hope with and for the good of those for whom they care.

Kubler-Ross' work showed not only the importance of hope in medicine and need for medical professionals to hope with and for those they care for. It also showed that the Percival tradition was wrong in its manner of sustaining this hope. Hope was not sustained by deception or lies. It was sustained by honesty. It was

---

[31] Ibid. pp. 22–23.
[32] Ibid. p. 23.
[33] Ibid. pp. 23–24.

sustained by listening to the patient and learning from him or her about their hopes, joys, anxieties, and fears. These are the parts of caretaking on which the patient is the expert and the physician or other caretakers the student.

V

At the end of the nineteenth century and into the early decades of the twentieth the connection between medicine, religion, and hope was given a strong new voice, fundamentally different than the "Percival tradition" we have been examining, by Richard Clarke Cabot. Cabot was a Harvard trained physician who wrote a great deal on medicine, the social sources of disease, and medical ethics. For example, he wrote a strong argument against the view of the tradition from Percival on defending honesty in medicine.[34]

In his pathbreaking view the care of the patient as a whole person was the responsibility of four professions: the doctor, the nurse, the social worker, and the minister, though the last category must include Jewish rabbis, Catholic priests, and other religious leaders.

These four professions collaborated to help the whole person recover their health. Persons are physical beings, which the physician and the nurse care for. They are also social beings, a truth as old in western thought as Aristotle. The social worker cares for and tries to heal their social situation. Finally, persons are spiritual beings, even if persons are reluctant to deal with these concerns. The "minister", broadly conceived, is the professional who can care for the spiritual life of the patient as a whole person.[35]

Cabot was a pioneer in many respects. A lasting effect of his work, however, was his creation of the social work department at Massachusetts General Hospital, the first of its kind in the United States. Because at first the hospital refused to fund social workers Cabot payed for them out of his own pocket. He also wrote extensively on ethics and was eventually appointed as professor of social ethics at Harvard.

His creation of medical social work as a profession was rooted in his belief that a person's health or illness was intrinsically connected to his or her whole life: living conditions, nutrition, employment, or lack thereof, etc. For examples: a man breaks his leg falling down stairs. Did he fall because the stairs were unsafe, and the owner of the apartment building refused to have them fixed? A woman gets a serious bacterial infection. Why? Because she is living in completely unsanitary conditions.

---

[34] Chester Burns, "Richard Clarke Cabot and the Revolution in American Medical Ethics". *Bulletin of the History of Medicine* 51(1977): 353–368; Laurie O'Brien "A Bold Plunge into a Sea of Values: The Career of Richard Clarke Cabot" *New England Quarterly* 58(1985): 333–353.

[35] Richard Clarke Cabot, "The Use of Truth and Falsehood in Medicine" *American Medicine* 5 (1903):344–349.

A person is very malnourished because they were fired from their job when they tried to form a union and demand better wages.[36]

In a passage that is very farsighted he writes: "The importance of social, psychical, and educational causes looms up larger and larger every year. Disease is not often 'hard luck' nor 'too bad'. For the most part it is as bad as we the taxpayers allow it to be—the unconquerable soul of us—recognize it to be. Preventable disease stares us in the face. Still the rank and file of the medical profession are too busy with cases of disease to have time for causes".[37]

Unlike Percival who was a Scottish Calvinist and the early AMA that represented those of various faiths or no faith, Cabot was a classic New England Unitarian. His parents were closely associated with the "transcendentalist" movement that involved Ralph Waldo Emerson, Henry David Thoreau, Margaret Fuller, F.H. Hedge, and Brooks Alcott. Even though his faith was liberal he believed that nourishing the spirit of the sick was as important as healing the body in helping the whole person recover their health. Without recognizing and treating these ills of the mind and spirit, it is impossible to relieve the bodily sufferings for which people consult the doctor. He lists these "moral and spiritual problems…doubt, fear, worry, remorse."

Furthermore, we note that in the distresses Cabot identifies and hundreds of others that could be cited, hope is essential to a person getting well. Rest and a vacation may relieve worry for a time. But these are diversions. Long term relief must be rooted in hope for a future with less persistent and profound worry, suffering or pain.

In this sense the doctor, nurse, social worker, and minister hope with the person who is sick, as Cabot would say, in both body and spirit. These professionals do not hope against the person, and they only partially hope for the person. They more deeply hope with person for the triumph of the good, for his or her good, that this person will emerge from their situation even in the darkest and most worrisome situation; that he will find a new and better job; that she will have more healthy food, and a warmer place to stay on cold nights. Finally, that this person can know that there is a power in the universe that brings about good.

Cabot states directly that when a person gets sick they should send for their minister just as they send for their doctor. Why must this be so? The minister has a special privilege that "springs from the fact that he has a living and sometimes contagious belief in God, in immortality and in the saving qualities of the gospel of Jesus Christ and in the soul's endless power of growth".[38]

The minister has a special, even revered, place in the care of the sick, because "mental and spiritual food is a crying need" which the minister is most adept at supplying. Doctors have neither the time nor the training to attend to the spiritual care

---

[36] Richard Clarke Cabot, *Social Service and the Art of Healing.* (New York: Moffitt and Company, 1914); Richard Clarke Cabot, *Social Work: Essays on the Meeting Ground of Doctor and Social Worker.* (Boston: Houghton Mifflin,19); Richard Clarke Cabot, "What's Worthwhile in Nursing?" *American Journal of Nursing.* 31(1931):277–285; Richard Clarke Cabot and Russel L. Dicks, *The Art of Ministering to the Sick.* (New York: Macmillan Company, 1936).

[37] Cabot, *Social Service and the Art of Healing,* op. cit. p. 36.

[38] Cabot and Dicks op. cit. p. 5.

of the sick nor to their social welfare. As such the minister and the social worker must be seen as essential partners in treating the whole person who is sick, not just a part of the person.

Patients are burdened with fear, apprehension, lack of confidence, lack of hope, and worries about his or her future, their family, their employment. True health relates to all of these concerns and the minister must be aware, as the doctor also. But the minister's special gift is to nourish the soul of the sick person and help the soul to grow by helping the sick person to realize that the "ground of his or her being is in God."

Patients are full persons, not just patients with physical ailments. In Percival's time, when medicine was not nearly as complicated as it was in Cabot's, the physician might have been able to play both roles. In Cabot's day, and much more so in ours, this was not possible.

What sick persons needed most was hope. First thing they needed was hope that they would get well: that they would return to work, to school, to household duties, to caring for their children, to making love to their spouse. Secondly, they needed hope in the face of the deepest fear of all: the fear of death. But Cabot reminds us, "to fear extinction is to distrust God" Jesus' "confidence was so strong that his followers caught it…the keynote of his life, his teaching, his influence is confidence in God. Whatever else he was, he was not fearful."

This confidence is not that of rational calculation. It is not based empirical probabilities rooted in a scientific understanding of the world and the patient's illness. This confidence rests on the hope that there is a power in the universe that makes for good.

Cabot was also a pioneer in another crucial part of medical ethics, lying to the patient. As we have seen, Percival and much of the tradition that came after him believed in what we can charitably refer to as "the benevolent lie" This practice was grounded in the belief that since the hope of the patient that he or she will get well was essential to their actually getting well, this hope should be sustained by the physician in every way possible. Either the physician should regularly tell the patient he or she will recover, when the physician believes otherwise or, at minimum, the physician should say nothing to discourage the patient's belief that they will recover.

Cabot deeply disagreed with this tradition. In a work published shortly before his death, *Honesty*, he harshly criticizes this and other "benevolent lies" and the crude moral utilitarianism that underlies such a view. He puts his point at exactly where he shows the error of such simplistic views as utilitarianism, situationism, an unthinking compassion as rationales for lying "Is not lying one of the greatest curses of the human race today." In this work he writes of the problem of lying and honesty in a number of fields, e.g., government, business, religion.[39]

---

[39] Richard Clarke Cabot, *Honesty*. (New York: Macmillan, 1938).

In an important chapter he writes of honesty in his own profession, medicine. To begin with he distinguishes physician honesty from physician infallibility. The former concerns whether the physician is honest with patient about what the physician believes is the correct diagnosis, treatment, and prognosis. The latter concerns whether the diagnosis and possible course of treatment are correct. Put another way, the first concerns honesty, the second concerns accuracy.

For Cabot dishonesty does not ultimately sustain hope. It undermines it. The physician who makes it a practice to never tell a truth that will supposedly undermine the patient's hope, soon finds that he must lie regularly If he or she only speaks the truth when it is good news will find that patients will never need to hope. Every day will be sunshine and flowers. Since every person knows that the world is not like that, patients will lose trust in their doctor who will not hope with them for improvement, nor will they know when to seek the comfort of a minister, priest, or rabbi.[40]

VI

Since the late 1950s codes of medical ethics by various medical associations have adopted the position of Cabot on the central question of truth telling in the doctor and patient relationship. The American Medical Association, the American College of Physicians, and other groups have stressed the right of the patient to know the truth about their medical condition no matter how unsettling or possibly fatal the condition maybe.[41]

Unfortunately, these codes and statements of principles have ignored the best part of the Percival on the importance of hope for a future good for the patient and others. They have adopted one of the best parts of the critique of the Percival tradition, but they have ignored another crucial part of Cabot's views that the whole person that medicine must treat including the social situation and the spiritual convictions of the patient and his family.

A couple of examples.

In the code from the American College of Physician we read patients "have a right to know what is in their medical record".[42]

---

[40] Richard Clarke Cabot, *Adventures on the Borderlands of Ethics*. (New York: Harper and Brothers, 1926).

[41] O. Wagsteen, "Should Patients be told they have Cancer?" *Surgery* 27(1950): 944–947; Donald Capon, "Attitudes of and Toward the Dying," *Canadian Medical Association Journal* 29(1952): 693–700; Eric Easson, "Cancer and the problem of Pessimism" *CA—Cancer* 17(1967): 7–14; Adrian Verwoerdt and Debby Wilson, "Communication with Terminally Ill Patients" *American Journal of Nursing* 67(1967): 2307–2309.

[42] American College of Physicians, *Ethics Manual*. Online https://doi.org/10.7326/m18-2160

The most recent text from the American medical association states: "patients have a right to receive information and ask questions about recommended treatments so that they can make well consider decisions about care. Successful communication in the patient physician relationship furthers trust and supports shared decision making".[43]

Since the 1960s the importance of informed consent has become central in medical care. Patient must give consent for any medical care. This principle is found in every code of medical ethics and is enshrined in government sponsored commissions and reports.[44] Except in emergency situations patients must give consent for the doctor's care. Patients cannot give informed consent without knowing what they are consenting to or rejecting.

Modern medicine has properly rejected the Percival tradition's belief in deception. But it has also downplayed the importance of sustaining the hope of the patient that good will triumphs over sickness, suffering, and possibly even death.

---

[43] American Medical Association, Code of Medical Ethics, *Shared Decision-Making*. Online at edhub.ama-assn.org

[44] The Belmont Report. *National Commission for the Protection of Human Subjects in Biomedical and Behavioral Research*. 1979; "Making Healthcare Decisions". *President's Commission for the Study of Ethical Problems in Medicine and Biomedical and Behavioral Research*. 1982.

Chapter 2
Epistemic Uncertainty

As we have seen in the first chapter and will see in more detail Chap. 4 hope is what humans have when certainty or high probability is lacking. I do not hope that the sun will set in the west at a precise time tomorrow evening. Given the likelihood that there will be stormy weather I can hope that I will see the sun in the morning.

If there will be cold weather, I can hope that my cherries and tomatoes will not freeze. But if the temperature goes down to 10 degrees Fahrenheit, I should not hope that the water in the bucket outside will not freeze. It will.

I do not hope that a human person needs to breathe to live. I can hope that an unconscious person in my driveway is still breathing or can be brought back to breathing with CPR. When the weather service predicts that there will be heavy rain in the morning, I can hope that the rain will not be as heavy as predicted or that it will not adversely affect my morning commute.

I Can the Doctor Achieve What he Knows is Right

In medicine uncertainty comes in two forms. The first form, the subject of this chapter, is what I call noetic or epistemic uncertainty. In these cases, the physician knows what the proper or right goal of his or her treatment should be: fix the crushed leg of the person so he or she can walk again; perform quadruple bypass surgery in a very difficult situation so the person can play golf or tennis again; or, with surgery and chemotherapy rid the woman's body of ovarian cancer.

In these cases, the uncertainty is not about knowing what the good result or goal of treatment is. The uncertainty is whether the medical professionals can actually achieve this goal. How much relief from heart problems can be achieved with bypass surgery; given that the ovarian cancer is stage 4 can the woman's life really be saved from her cancer. Since the leg has been broken in four places from an auto accident can this person walk again without braces, crutches, or a walker?

The second form of uncertainty is what I refer to as moral uncertainty. In this sort of case the physician knows or is reasonably certain what he or she can do but is very uncertain whether they should do it. Suppose a male patient wants to have his testicles removed so that he will be able to stop thinking about having sexual intercourse with underage girls. The doctor knows what he can do. The surgery is not difficult. It has an almost 100% success rate. But should he deliberately maim a person?

In another case a woman comes to her doctor for a medical check-up, including a mammogram. The mammogram and the physician's hand touch reveal the possibility of a breast tumor. What is first required to study this further is a biopsy of what appears to be a tumor. This is an easy procedure and will not take more than 2 hours in the hospital. But the patient will not permit it. She believes that if air gets on the tumor, it will spread and lead to her death. She lives her life without mental problems. She is not incompetent. Here, as before, the physician knows what right goal is. However, he or she is deeply uncertain about how to achieve it. These sorts of cases are the subject of the next chapter.

II Cases

Let us now examine four cases where this sort of epistemic uncertainty is exemplified.

Charles (Chuck)

Charles Gardner is a successful 45 year old tax attorney in city of half a million people. He focuses his work on medium sized businesses of 50–100 employees. He handles all of their federal, state, and local taxes, He also handles their property taxes. He establishes tax withholding, including workman's compensation and quarterly and annual filings. If either state or federal tax officials have questions about the filings, he handles all the inquiries.

Chuck has been happily married for 25 years to a woman he met in college, Joan. Chuck and Joan have four children. One is a sophomore in college, two are in high school and the last is in 7th grade. Joan works part time as a school nurse. Chuck and Joan are active in their evangelical church. Chuck does the taxes for the pastor and his wife free of charge.

For several weeks Chuck has had problems with his urination. The urinary stream has been very week and he has had to get up several times during the night to urinate. His father had to get up several times during the night to urinate. But that was when his father was in his early 70s. This is common. As men age their prostate enlarges and pushes on their bladder. As such, the bladder cannot hold as much urine as it did when the man was younger. This enlargement is not due to cancer. It is a natural consequence of aging.

Chuck makes an appointment with the family's primary care physician, Dr. Mark Linden. Dr. Linden gives Chuck both a physical examination of his prostate and draws blood for a prostate specific antigen (PSA) test for prostate cancer. Both tests show that Chuck has prostate cancer. Dr. Linden refers Chuck to a urologist who has an office in the same building, Dr. Fred Frazier. Dr. Frazier has wide experience with prostate cancer. Dr. Frazier confirms the diagnosis. With more tests he determines how advanced the cancer is and what the treatment options are. Dr. Frazier schedules an appointment for Chuck and his wife Joan. Chuck informs his pastor who prays for him and asks the congregation to pray for Chuck and Joan.[1]

Dr. Frazier informs Chuck and Joan that the cancer has, very likely, not spread outside of the prostate He also informs them that radical surgical removal of the entire prostate and surrounding tissue is the best option. This option will best ensure the complete removal of the cancer such that it will not return.

In his treatment of Chuck and Joan Dr. Frazier has three goals. The first is to completely remove the cancer so that it will not return later. The second is to preserve and improve Chuck's urinary continence so that Chuck will not need a catheter and a urinary bag. Thirdly, Dr. Frazier would like to preserve Chuck's ability to sustain an erection so that Chuck and Joan can enjoy a satisfying intimate life. Chuck and Joan have a strong marriage and they are only in their early 40s. A satisfying sex life is important to them.

Dr. Frazier has these three goals. But achieving all of them equally well will be very difficult. Complete removal of the prostate is the best option to ensure that cancer is gone and will not return. This option, however, will severely affect Chuck's ability to have sexual intimacy with Joan. Some types of surgery may affect his urinary continence. In short, Dr. Frazier must hope that his treatment of Chuck and his wife will have a positive result.

Margaret Dolan

Margaret Dolan has been mentally unstable for many months. Many days she has trouble just getting out of bed. She lays in bed just watching anything on TV, without much care what the program is She does not eat well and when she eats, she

---

[1] On prostate cancer: Andrew Siegal, *Prostate Cancer 20/20: A practical Guide to Understanding, Management, and Treatment Options for Patients and their Families.* (Louisville: Rogue Wave, 2019); Harley Haynes and Richard Miles, *The Prostate Cancer Owners Manuel: Want You Need to Know About Diagnosis, Treatment and Survival* (Baltimore: Rowman and Littlefield, 2021); John Mulhall, *Saving Your Sex Life: A Guide for Men with Prostate Cancer.* (Chicago: Hilton, 2008); Ralph Allenowitz and Barbara Allenowitz, *Intimacy with Impotence: A Couples Guide to Better Sex After Prostate Disease.* (Boston: Da Capo, 2004).

often over eats. She has gained a substantial amount of weight. Some days she feels so sad that she has considered suicide.

Her husband, Don, has finally convinced her to see their family physician as have their grown children. Dr. Granger, the family physician, easily diagnoses severe depression and prescribes Paxil, a well-known SSRI (selective serotonin reuptake inhibitor)[2] Dr. Granger refers her to a nearby mental health clinic for follow-up treatment. Don makes the appointment for her at the clinic and accompanies her to insure she goes.

At the clinic she starts seeing Martha Davis, a counselor, every week, and she sees Dr. George Henkson, a psychiatrist, for medication follow-up. After about 4 months on Paxil, her depression has lifted. Don sees the woman he fell in love with decades earlier. Now, however, a new problem arises. Margaret is having trouble sleeping. She wants to be doing something, anything, all the time. At times she starts believing that the newscaster on the local television station is talking directly to her.

Dr. Henkson easily recognizes the symptoms of serious mania. Mania is more than just being excited or happy most of the time. Sometimes some people do have difficulty sleeping for various reasons, even though they are not manic. But for Dr. Henkson the key is the belief that the newscaster is speaking directly to Margaret. For professionals such as Martha Davis and Dr. Henkson this is known as "referential thinking" or "referential delusions".[3] Dr. Henkson prescribes clonazepam for immediate relief and a widely used and effective mood stabilizer, Depakote, for long term treatment.[4]

After 6 weeks Margaret's mood has stabilized, her counselor says she is doing well. But serious side effects of the Depakote are starting to emerge: dizziness, fever, and stomach pain. Since Depakote has serious side effects, Dr. Henkson tapers her off it and starts her on another widely used mood stabilizer, Seroquel.[5] After about 5 weeks on Seroquel Margaret's mood has stabilized well. But now serious side effects, very similar to those of Depakote, start to appear: stomach cramps and fever especially, as well as often serious anxiety. Dr. Henkson tries adjusting her dosage to find one that can stabilize her mood with less or no side effects. As with Depakote, however, he is unable to achieve both of these goals as well as he and Margaret would like.

---

[2] Linda Fulton, *Hope: A Comprehensive Guide to Living with and Defeating Manic Depression.* (Create Space Publishing, 2016); Lana Castle, *Bipolar Disorder Demystified.* (Boston: Da Capo, 2007); E. Fuller Torrey and Michael Knoble *Surviving Manic Depression.* (New York: Basic Books, 2005); Kay Redfield Jameson An *Unquiet Mind: A Memoir of Moods and Madness.* (New York: Vintage, 1996).

[3] Seroquel (quetiapine) Web MD. Com.

[4] Depakote (divalproex) Web MD. Com.

[5] Harrington Rods were stainless steel rods that were implanted next to the spine to stabilize the spinal column and hold the vertebrae in place. They were widely used from the early 1950s to the mid 1990s.

Dr. Henkson knows that in manic depression psychotherapy, is only effective for two purposes. The therapist can. Encourage the patient to stay on medication and the therapist can give the psychiatrist a professional account of how the patient is doing and the possible need to adjust or change their medication. He also knows that in some persons manic depressive disorder is difficult to manage. This is especially true in rapid cycling manic depression, which appears to be the case for Margaret.

Since Seroquel and Depakote have too many bad side effects Dr. Henkson now tries the most widely used mood stabilizer, lithium. Lithium was explicitly used to treat manic depressive disorder after World War II and intermittently for centuries before that. Even in ancient times doctors would advise patients with mental disorders to drink water from alkali springs. Unknowingly they were prescribing lithium. Alkali springs are rich in lithium salts. Of course, there are side effects: gastrointestinal upset, sedation, frequent urination. Excessive blood lithium levels can cause kidney damage. Hence, careful monitoring is required, especially when starting lithium.[6]

After several months on lithium Margaret has been doing reasonably well. But she starts to cycle back into mania. She has trouble sleeping. She wants to buy things for the house they do not need. She also has to urinate very frequently. The manic episodes are less frequent. But mania has returned. For Dr. Henkson this seems to be a very difficult case. Margaret may always have cycles of depression and mania. Although less frequent than before, they will always be there.

Dr. Henkson knows what the goal in caring for Margaret is: stabilize her moods so that she can care for and with her husband, go shopping, go out with friends, go to a concert or dinner with Don. What Dr. Henkson does not know is whether this goal can be achieved. He, the counselor, Margaret, and Dan can only hope that this goal can be achieved.

Claire Darlington

Claire Darlington, a 49-year-old widowed woman with one son, has felt sick for several months. For her the sickness is over her whole body, not from any specific location such as a headache, bruised abdomen, or very sore neck. After several weeks her self administered ibuprofen and hot baths have had little effect. She goes to see her local internist, Dr. Jim Miller. He sees she is depressed and starts her on Celexa, a well-known SSRI. Her mood does improve. But this does nothing to improve her feeling sick all over her body. He prescribes antibiotics, bed rest, and nutritional supplements. He also has blood tests and urinalysis as well as a CT scan at a local hospital. The blood work showed that she had systemic infection, but no source was discovered.

---

[6] Stephen Kirshblum and Vernon Lin, *Spinal Cord Medicine* 3rd ed. (Demos Medical, 2018); J. Kalyvas and N. Theodore "Lumbar Spine Stabilization" in Michael Aminoff and Robert Doroff eds. *Encyclopedia of the Neurological Sciences* (Amsterdam: Elsevier, 2004).

After several weeks her health was getting much worse. Dr. Miller has her airlifted to the hospital at a major university medical school 90 miles away where she can be examined by specialists. At the hospital she is again found to have low blood pressure, labored breathing, and difficulty urinating. Her abdomen is very tender to the touch. She feels sick throughout her body. She has limited kidney function and her liver and pancreas are inflamed. The hospital's (and medical school's) infectious disease specialist Dr. Karen Steel examines her carefully as do a kidney specialist and a pulmonary specialist.

After these examinations, Dr. Steel asks her brothers to call all the family and friends together as soon as possible. She informs Claire's family and friends that Claire will very likely die that night. She is too ill and too much infected throughout her body to survive much longer.

Claire's family are very religious. They engage in deep prayer for her life. The priest in her hometown is contacted. He puts them in touch with the university's Newman Center whose priests cover the university hospital as well as its children's hospital. Father Dansie from the Newman Center comes quickly and performs the Sacrament of Anointing the Sick, what used to be informally called "last rites".[7] He prays with and for the family. He tells the family to call him, even in the middle of the night, if anything changes. At daily mass in her hometown that night the priest includes her in "the prayers of the faithful" which are also called "intercessions".

In the morning, almost "miraculously", Claire has not died. She is still expected to die almost at any moment. A surgeon, Dr. Gupta, and Dr. Steel come to talk to Claire's brothers. They are the only family able understand the situation and to give consent for any further treatment. Dr. Gupta and Dr. Steel inform the brothers that the only chance for Claire's survival is to find the source of Claire's infection and remove it. The surgery will be long and difficult. Dr. Gupta tells the family that Claire's chances of surviving the operation are very slim. She will very likely die during surgery. This surgery, however, is the only possible course to save Claire's life.

Dr. Gupta and Dr. Steel know what the right goal of their treatment is: find the source of the infection and remove it. They have no doubt about this goal. They are, however, deeply uncertain about whether they can achieve this goal. Dr. Steel expected her death during the night. They expect her death in surgery. What they can do is "hope against hope" that Claire's life can be saved.

Dan Kelly

Dan Kelly is a 45-year-old happily married man who owns a prosperous automobile repair shop in a city of about 200,000. Dan and his wife Sue have three children. Two are graduates of the local state college. The third is still in college studying to

---

[7] Albert Camus, *The Plague*. trans. Stuart Gilbert (New York: Alfred Knopf, 1948).

II Cases

be a high school English teacher. He and Sue's oldest son is married with one grandchild.

While painting the trim on his house Dan falls off the ladder and his back hits squarely on a large rock. He immediately recognizes that he has been seriously injured. He is in great pain, and he has trouble standing and walking. Believing that bed rest, ibuprofen, and a heating pad will be successful in restoring his health, He rests the rest of that day and the next. The ibuprofen and the heating pad help, but great pain remains.

With Sue's help he goes to see their family doctor Lee Martin. Doctor Martin prescribes a narcotic analgesic (Percocet) for better pain relief and refers Dan to an orthopedic specialist for a more thorough examination and treatment.

Dr. Laurence Wilson, the orthopedic specialist recognizes that Dan has severe trauma at the T-6 area of his spine. Dr. Wilson brings in as part of his care team Dr. Paul Flandro a neurosurgeon with a specialty in spinal surgery. After a physical examination and CT scans they conclude that given the severity of the spinal trauma spinal surgery is the best treatment option. The spinal column is not ruptured but it is badly bruised, and two vertebrae are displaced. Surgical repair of displaced vertebrae and stabilization of the spine with "Harrington rods" is the best option.[8] Dr.'s Wilson and Flando inform Dan and his wife of their evaluation and recommendation. Bed rest, heating pads, relaxation will be ineffective. Narcotic analgesics will only mask the symptoms and be highly addictive. Steroids to relieve the spinal swelling offer little permanent relief and are rarely used anymore for these sorts of cases. Neck or spinal braces offer some temporary help but, again, they do not treat the underlying cause. The doctors also inform Dan and Sue that substantial data show that the sooner surgery is performed in these sorts of cases the better the outcome.

Since Dr. Flandro has much more experience in spinal surgery, he will perform the surgery and Dr. Wilson will assist. Dr. Flandro has four goals of his treatment of Dan. First, he wants to relieve the source of the severe spinal stress and pain that Dan has, so he will not need narcotic painkillers and try to get them by doctor shopping or even illegally. Secondly, he wants to preserve as much as possible Dan's physical mobility so that he can walk and mow the lawn. Almost certainly Dan will not be able to play tennis. But Dr. Flandro would like him to be able to walk around the block. Thirdly Dr. Flandro would like to preserve, as much as possible Dan's urinary continence so that he will not need a catheter and a urinary bag. Finally, he would like to preserve Dan's ability to sustain an erection and maintain a satisfying sex life with Sue, his wife of 25 years. Since they are only in their mid-40s and they have a strong marriage, this intimacy is important for them.

Dr. Flandro is highly certain that he can relieve the pressure on the spine which is causing the severe pain. He is also relatively certain that he can succeed in preserving Dan's physical mobility. He is less certain about fully sustaining Dan's urinary continence. When pressed by Dan and Sue he estimates that the likelihood of

---

[8] *Plague* p. 7.

preserving Dan's continence as 50/50. Finally, he regards it as very unlikely that ne can preserve Dan's ability to sustain an erection and have that sort of intimate life with Sue. This is especially true in light of the radical surgery required to relieve the stress on his spine. What Dr. Flandro, Dan and Sue must do is hope that these goals, that are themselves good, can be achieved.

III   The Plague

One of the greatest novels of the twentieth century is also a wonderful story of this sort of medical uncertainty and the importance of hope in the face of sickness, suffering, and death. The novel is Albert Camus' classic *The Plague* (La Peste). It is set in Camus' hometown, Oran, in French Algeria sometime in the late 1940s.[9]

The major characters are:

Dr. Bernard Rieux—An atheist physician
Father Paneloux—A Catholic priest
M. Mercier—A local public official
Joseph Grand—An elderly man
Dr. Richard, a more cautious physician
Dr. Castel—Am elderly physician who has a small medical laboratory.

"One morning after leaving his surgery" Dr. Rieux steps on a dead rat on the landing of his building. The date is April 16. He thought nothing of it until he reached the street. There should not have been a dead rat in the building was his thought.[10]

In the following days more dead rats kept piling up where they should not have been found. At this point, however, no one is really alarmed. Rieux's wife has dressed up for a vacation. He sees her off at the train station. She asks him about the stories circulating about dead rats. He says he can't explain it. "But it will pass" he tells her. He is not worried.[11]

Dead rats, however, keep piling up. On April 18 Mercier, the public official, found 50 dead rats in his office,[12] After the 18th dead rats were piling up everywhere in the city and surrounding suburbs. Trash cans were filling up every day. The public was getting very worried daily. By April 28, 8000 dead rats had been found so far. On that date M. Michel, the concierge in Rieux's building became very sick in the street and had to be almost carried to Dr. Rieux by Father Paneloux, "a learned and militant Jesuit."[13] On that same day an elderly man almost hung himself because of his fear and sadness about what was happening. On April 30, only 2 weeks after the

---

[9] *Plague* p. 10.
[10] *Plague* p. 14.
[11] *Plague* p. 17.
[12] Ibid.
[13] *Plague* p. 36.

III The Plague

first dead rat, M. Michel died of whatever it was causing the death and destruction that was striking Oran.[14]

People were getting sick and dying every day. The sickness and death toll were increasing at an alarming rate every day. The papers, however, were silent about the rising death toll. They did not want to further terrify an already terrified population. Silence, the editors thought, was better than the truth. Perhaps a slightly different version of the Percival tradition.[15]

Dr. Castel, one of Rieux's friends and colleagues, though much older, comes to see him. "You know what it is" Castel told him. Rieux professed not to know until further investigations were completed. Castel stopped him. "I know and I don't need tests or to wait further". Castel had been in China for many years and had seen cases just like this in Paris in the 1920s. In Paris, however, no one dared to tell the truth for fear of causing a panic in the population. After a minute Rieux admits the truth of what Castel knows "everything points to it being the plague".[16]

A meeting of doctors and public officials is called. Some doctors profess not to know. They want more tests and more cases. Castel and Rieux are sure. They argue that the doctors and city officials cannot wait to take drastic measures to protect the public. Others, like those in Paris 20 years before don't want to create a panic. Rieux makes his point powerfully "we should not act as if there were no likelihood that half the population would be wiped out, for then it would be." If they don't act as if many will die, many will.[17]

Unfortunately, there was no "serum" to treat the plague in the area. A telegram was sent to Paris to have them send "serum" Some "serum" arrived by plane the next day. "Enough for Immediate requirements". But not enough if the epidemic were to spread of get worse. In Paris the emergency supply was exhausted. Oran was told that more was being prepared but it was unknown how long it would take for Oran to receive more.[18]

Now drastic measures were finally being taken. The city gates were closed. No one could enter or leave. No planes, trains, buses, or cars could come or go. No one could go and see loved ones or wives. Rieux's wife could not return to be with him. Children could not visit aging parents. Nor could parents see grandchildren. Even mail could not be sent because of fear that this could spread the disease. Only telegrams could be sent or received. The plague had almost completely isolated the city and its people.[19]

Since no planes could fly in no more serum could be flown in from Paris. This meant that the city, its people, and its doctors must "fend for themselves" In short, they must hope for relief from their suffering with little certainty that any relief will

---

[14] *Plague* p. 51.

[15] *Plague* pp. 67–70.

[16] *Plague* pp. 97–99.

[17] *Plague* pp. 211–217.

[18] *Plaque* pp. 192–193.

[19] *Plague* p. 255.

come before, perhaps, half the citizens do die from the plague. Before the pandemic on Sundays the beaches were full and the churches almost empty. Now the beaches are deserted, and Father Paneloux has standing room only.

As hotter weather set in deaths increased, averaging about 700 a week. No one enjoyed much of anything. Schools had been taken over as makeshift hospitals. The plague had "killed all colors, vetoed pleasure". Fear was pervasive. Even if the sky was blue and the weather warm, the souls of the citizens and the city itself were dark and terrified.

Castel, with most experience with the plague set up a makeshift lab and spent every moment he had to develop a serum to relieve the suffering of the people of Oran. The suffering, the seeming hopelessness, the darkness of the souls, and the future carried on for weeks which turned into months. Finally, at the end of October, a little over 5 months after the beginning of the plague, (both symbolic and real) Castel's serum is ready to try for the first time.

A young boy who has just fallen ill was selected as the first person on which to test the serum. M. Othon and his wife Madame Othon want their son to live. "Save my son" she cries. The boy was taken to an auxiliary hospital that had once been a school. Rieux thought the likelihood of success was low, but he had "no qualms about testing Castel's 'serum' on the boy". Yet Rieux cannot have believed that the situation was without any hope. If he really believed this, why try. One does not try to resuscitate a dead body.

If the "serum" works, the city can breathe a sigh of relief. If it does not work, the citizens can still hope for relief. But this "serum" will not be the answer. What about the young boy, however? What if it only prolongs his dying and does not prevent it? Father Paneloux, who is there, states the truth "so if he is to die, he will have suffered longer." In the end, as the boy is suffering, Paneloux sinks to his knees and cries out "My God, save this child" The boy dies after having suffered longer.

After the ordeal is over Rieux and Paneloux talk. As Paneloux notes they are both "working for man's salvation". One for the health of the body, one for the health of the soul. What unites them is that they must hope for the good to triumph over human suffering a good of body and soul. They must hope that even in suffering good can emerge. Even in the boy's death Castel might have learned how to improve his serum. That the Othons might have gained a greater faith in a life for their son beyond the grave.

Throughout this story hope is at the center of belief and action. Rieux must hope that the first dead rat is not a sign of something worse. Other doctors hope that the sickness is not the plague. When Castel and Rieux convince them that it is, they all hope that it will soon pass, that Rieux was right in what he told his wife as she boarded the train.

When Castel's serum is ready to try the boy's parents hope that it will save their son. If it will not, they must hope that he will not suffer longer. All the citizens, parents, children, doctors, and Father Paneloux know what the right goal is: relieve the suffering and death of the citizens of Oran. They must hope that this goal can be achieved, the sooner the better. They have no way of knowing when or how it will happen.

IV Examinig the Cases

The four cases we started with are actual examples that I know personally. They exemplify hope in medicine, epistemic hope. In these cases, the doctor knows, in a broad sense of knowing, what the right goal or goals of treatment are. He or she knows what they should achieve with this person or couple. The doctor, however, is profoundly uncertain, whether this goal or goals can be the result of the treatment that the doctor knows is right. Thus, the doctor cannot know that what is good can come from the treatment of this person. They and the person being treated must hope.

Two of these cases have one primary goal. Save Claire's life so she can work and raise her son. Stabilize Margaret's mood so she can have a reasonably normal life with her husband of 25 years. The other two cases are where there is more than one goal of treatment, goals that are themselves good. Chuck and Joan have a very good marriage. They are relatively young and sexual intimacy as a married couple is important to them as it is to most married couples in their age range. Thus, along with removing Chuck's cancer, this is an important goal for Chuck and Joan. This also is one of the important goals in the treatment of Dan and Sue who are also relatively young and have a good marriage. Though the primary goal of the treatment of both Chuck and Dan is different, the other goals are similar. Like Dr. Rieux each of the doctors in these four cases know what the goal of treatment is. They must hope that they can achieve these goals.

Margaret's case is typical of rapid cycling manic depression, what is also called bi-polar disorder. Anti-depressive medications, especially SSRI's, have been a real blessing for those who suffer from serious depression. They have enabled millions to lead healthy, relatively normal lives. It turns out that the most effective treatment for severe depression is medication and cognitive therapy. Just the sort of treatment Margaret is able to receive at the community mental health center.

Manic depression is fundamentally different. Though in Margaret's case it becomes serious at a later age, in her 40s, than it typically does in someone's 20s. In manic depression successfully treating the depression is only part of the battle. With medication and talk therapy, it is often the most successful. This was the case in Margaret's treatment at the community mental health center.

What is often much more difficult is reducing, managing, or even eliminating the manic episodes. As it is in Margaret's case this is often much more difficult to achieve in manic depression. This is especially true in persons like Margaret with rapid cycling manic depressive disorder.

Dr. Henkson finds Margaret's manic-depressive disorder difficult to manage. He can and does successfully treat her depression with Paxil a well-known SSRI. What is difficult, however, as it is in many cases of manic depression, is stabilizing her mood so that serious manic episodes do not happen or happen very infrequently.

Dr. Henkson's goal is to find the right dose or combinations of mood stabilizers and an SSRI to achieve the result that he, Margaret, and Margaret's husband Don, know is the right result. An SSRI and Martha Davis' therapy can successfully treat her depression. As in many cases of manic depression, like Margaret's, stabilizing her mood will be difficult and uncertain. Dr. Henkson does not and cannot know whether he will be able to do this successfully. Dr. Henkson, Margaret and Don must hope that in her case good triumphs over sickness and suffering.

At least in Margaret's case, with treatment for depression, she is not likely to die from her illness or commit suicide. This is not the case with Claire's sickness. Claire has been very sick for months. Her son has tried to help her as have her friends. When she was hospitalized for tests in her hometown, friends cared for her son. Antidepressants and counseling have relieved partially the depression that has accompanied her illness. But this care has not relieved her sickness all over her body. What is needed is to find the source of her systemic infection and remove or treat that, not just treat the recurring symptoms.

Dr.'s Gupta and Steel know what the right goal is. Of this they have no doubt: save Claire's life. To achieve this goal, they must find the source of her sickness and successfully treat it. Without finding the source and treating or removing it Claire will die. The doctors thought that she would have died already. They know that something inside of Claire's body is the source of her sickness and suffering. Thus, surgery is the only possibility for saving her life. Dr. Gupta believes that the likelihood of success of surgery is very low. But he is willing to do what he can and must do to save Claire's life. In short Dr. Gupta must hope that Claire's life can be saved.

Claire's family are very religious. Given their faith it is entirely reasonable for them to pray for divine intervention and to ask friends and fellow congregants to pray for a "miracle". Dr. Steel is religious but not of Claire's specific faith, though she is a believing Christian. As Christians Claire, her family, and Dr. Steel can and do hope that Claire's life, will be saved, that God will bring about good, even though they do not and cannot know how or when.

But Claire is not dead. Dr.'s Gupta and Steel must hope, even "hope against hope" that they can save Claire's life. Without this hope they cannot act to save her life. They must hope with and for her family, friends, priest, fellow congregants, and son that her life will not end on the operating table.

The cases of Charles Gardner and Dan Kelly are different in one major way and several smaller ones. The most crucial difference is that for Claire and Margaret there is one primary goal in each case: save Claire's life, stabilize Margaret's mood. In the cases of Chuck and Dan there is more than one goal in each case. This fact makes it more difficult for the doctor in each case to be able to fully achieve all the goals they know are right in each case.

Chuck is a healthy early middle-aged man with a strong marriage, wonderful family, deep religious faith, and a prosperous career. Prostate cancer has disrupted his and his family's life in a serious way. Of course, his, his family's and Dr. Frazier's primary goal is to preserve his life and do so in a permanent way. None of them want the cancer to return or to spread elsewhere in Chuck's body.

Almost as important is Chuck's strong marriage to Joan. Chuck wants to make physical love to his wife as married couple do at their age. This part of their lives is important to them, and they desire that it continues. As a doctor who has treated many cases of prostate cancer, especially couples in the age range of Chuck and Joan, Dr. Frazier knows how important this is for couples like them. After talking extensively with them he knows specifically how important this is to Chuck and Joan specifically.

Chuck's continence is also important. His uncle had to have a catheter and urinary bag for several years so Chuck knows first-hand how bothersome such a result can be to manage on a practical basis. There are parts of your life that it affects on a daily basis. With a catheter and a bag, the person has to be constantly aware of the placement of the catheter and how much urine is in the bag. The person must be sure that the bag is fully emptied properly and that none spills in the office, on the bathroom floor, or on the person's clothes.

These are practical matters that the person must be aware of constantly. The person must care for themselves well. They must watch their health better than they may have done in the past. Joan, of course, can be of great assistance in this regard. But Chuck is the person most affected by the possibility of a bag and catheter, so he must care for himself well and constantly.

For Chuck and Joan, however, aside from eliminating the cancer, their most important goal is to preserve the possibility of marital intimacy, even if it is not as frequent as before the cancer treatment. This desire is equally important for both Chuck and Joan. For Dr. Frazier it is also very important.

Dr. Frazier knows that the best way to ensure that the prostate cancer will be eliminated and never return is to completely remove the prostate and all surrounding tissue. He also knows that this treatment will eliminate any possibility of Chuck and Joan having the sexual intimacy they have had and want to have in the future. Dr. Frazier also knows that there are less radical surgical options that might preserve Chuck's ability for sexual intimacy with his wife. He also knows that these options are less certain to eliminate any possibility of the cancer returning.

What Dr. Frazier, Chuck and Joan must do is hope in several ways. Chuck and Joan must hope that if they choose the radical surgery, the option that will most certainly prevent the cancer from returning, that they can sustain their strong marriage, though sexual intimacy will not be part of it. If they choose an option that will preserve the possibility of marital intimacy, they and Dr. Frazier must hope that the cancer will not return.

Chuck, Joan, and Dr. Frazier know what the goals of treatment are. Of these goals they have no doubt. Nor should there be any doubt that these are good goals. What they must do is hope that these goals, especially removing the cancer and preserving the possibility of marital intimacy can be achieved.

Dan Kelly now knows that he should have had a professional do what he was doing, painting the trim on his house. A professional would have had a better ladder. The professional would also have insured that nothing near the ladder could have caused serious injury from a fall.

After finding out the nature and extent of his injuries from Dr.'s Wilson and Flandro, Dan knows that he will not be able to run 5K or 10K runs as he has done. Nor will he be able to play tennis like he has been doing for years, especially competitive doubles with his wife in a local league or just with friends as they do almost every week. But Dan would like to go on walks with his wife as they have done for years, even if the walks are not as long as they once were. Nor does he want to have to use a walker. It may take several months of recuperation and physical therapy to reach this goal. But Dan hopes that this goal can be reached.

Dan and Sue hope that Dan will not need a catheter and urinary bag. Dr. Flandro gives them a rough estimate of a 50/50 chance of not needing a bag. Dan and Sue hope that they will be on the positive side of the ledger, like the hope of Chuck and Joan. However, more important than the possibility of needing a catheter is their desire to sustain the possibility of sexual intimacy as a married couple. Dan and Sue have a strong marriage and a robust intimate life which is important to them as a married couple.

Dan's physical mobility is important to him. His assistants can maintain the business while he has surgery and a period of recuperation. His good mechanics can keep his customers satisfied with their repairs. But Dan is a "hands on" owner/manager. He likes to inspect the work of his mechanics so he can know that the work is done well. If a mechanic finds an unforeseen problem, Dan wants to see the problem himself so he can talk directly to the customer and explain the problem and the options for repair.

Dr. Flandro is very optimistic that he can restore Dan's physical mobility so he can walk around his business, his home, his neighborhood, and the mall without either a walker or a cane. Of course, this optimism is less certain than that the sun will rise at a specific time in the morning, so some hope is involved. Where hope enters this case directly is at two places. First, can Dan have urinary continence without a catheter and a bag. Secondly, for Dan and Sue their marital intimacy is important. Here hope is even more crucial. In cases like Dan's many persons have difficulty of having an erection. Many others cannot sustain an erection long enough to enjoy an intimate relation with their wife. After surgery and rehabilitation Dan will probably need to see a urologist who specializes in treating cases like this. If this part of their life is lost Dan and Sue will need to find other ways to sustain their marital intimacy; ways that they must hope can be successful.

Dr. Flandro can achieve his first two goal with and for Dan. The last two Dan, Sue and Dr. Flandro must hope that they can be achieved, if only imperfectly.

V

These cases are all real but appropriately changed for reasons of confidentiality and privacy. They are, however, only examples. Along with Dr's Rieux and Castel, they are examples of one form of hope in human caretaking. The caretaker, including but not limited to a doctor, must hope that good can come out of what is bad, wrong, or evil. The caretaker knows what the goal is. But he or she must hope that good will result from the care. The Othon's must hope that if their son is not saved by the "serum" that he can have a life beyond the grave. They cannot know this in the way that they can know that the earth revolves around the sun. They must hope because they cannot know.

V   33

The citizens of Oran can hope for relief, not knowing where or how it will come. They can hope that though in this trial Castel's "serum" was not successful, he may be able to improve it based on what he learned. They can hope that it will be successful next time. Atheist, scientist Dr. Rieux must hope that something good come out of his work, though science itself cannot justify this hope.

Rieux was exhausted. He was getting 4 hours of sleep every night. He constantly cared for the sick and the dying. His science could only take him so far. What these people needed was care, that included but went beyond science. A woman told him angrily, "You have no heart". She was wrong. As a human being and as a caretaker he had a generous heart. "It saw him through his twenty our days when he saw the dying who were meant to live. It enabled him to start anew each morning."

Though he is reluctant to admit it, his heart was rooted in a hope for the good that his medical training did not realize, and his atheism did not let him see clearly. His humanity and his caretaking brought him to this hope. When Tarrou asks the seminal question "Can you be a saint and an atheist?" Rieux's life is an answer: yes. Saints act for a good beyond themselves and beyond what they can rationally believe. Rieux doesn't believe in the god of western theism. But his heart must hope for a good he cannot see or know. He knows what the right goal of his care and Castel's serum must be. He, the other doctors, and the people of Oran must hope that this good can be reached.

The four cases are examples of what I have called epistemic hope. In each case there is little doubt about what the goal or goals are. The goal or goals are well understood, and they are not contested or controversial. In the cases of Chuck and Dan there is more than one goal so the person, his family, and the doctor must decide which of the three goals should come first. Or should the achievement of one goal be compromised so that another goal might be achieved. But this decision is not about whether two goals are good but about how to achieve them. It's not a moral judgment but an epistemic one.

Some of these persons, families and doctors are deeply religious in a western, monotheistic sense. Others are not. Yet each doctor, patient, and family must hope in a similar way. Chuck and Joan, Claire's family, and Dr. Steel can pray for divine intervention. Chuck's pastor and Claire's priest can pray with and for the patient and the family. Margaret's doctor is not religious in the traditional sense. These doctors as well as Margaret's and Dan's families must hope that the good can come out of this care. Even in Claire's case, Dr. Gupta would not try to save her life if there was no hope that this was possible. In each of these cases, as it is in the fictional world of Oran, hope is at the core human caretaking.

Chapter 3
Moral Uncertainty in Medicine

The first form of uncertainty in medicine was what I have called epistemic or noetic. This is focused on knowledge and technical skill. Can the doctor do what she knows, in a broad sense of know, should be the right result from her treatment of the patient? Dr. Gupta knows what the right result should be in his treatment of Ms. Darlington. He is profoundly uncertain about whether he can achieve this result. If he cannot, Claire will die sooner.

Bernard Rieux knows what he should do. He does not know whether he can. If he tries and fails, he may increase the suffering of the young boy. Without trying, however, no vaccine will be found.

The vastly increased knowledge and technical skill of modern medicine, which, as we noted, contributes highly to better diagnosis, also increases noetic uncertainty. Knowing what illness the patient has, diagnosis, has substantially increased beyond our ability to successfully treat many illnesses.

Increased knowledge and skill have also deeply affected the second, and probably more common, uncertainty in medicine: moral uncertainty. In these cases, the doctor knows what she is able to do, but is profoundly uncertain about whether she should do what she is able to do.

I Cases

Let us start, then, with some actual cases of this sort of uncertainty.

Vicki Cline

Vicki is a 30-year-old woman who is healthy, attractive, and hardworking. She graduated from college magna cum laude with a degree in accounting and spent an extra year in school specializing in tax accounting. Vicki now works for a major accounting firm in a large city, where she has just become a partner.

She has dated several men, but nothing has ultimately worked out. Though her romantic life has not gone as she had hoped, in every other way her life seems to be blessed.

Yet Vicki is deeply uneasy. For years she has been living with a condition known as aptomenophilia, also known as body integrity identity disorder.[1] In this condition Vicki has a deep feeling that the body she has is the not the body she is supposed to have. It is not that her body is abnormal in any way. She is physically fit, slender, and attractive.

Rather, in this condition she believes that she should have her left hand amputated. Then, she believes, her body will be "perfect". If it is amputated then it will be the body she believes she is meant to have.

She goes to see a well-regarded orthopedic surgeon in her city, Dr. Ellen Stayer. Dr. Stayer has seen this condition a couple of times before. Her first reaction is to have Vicki see a psychotherapist for mental health care. Though she knows that this sort of care is likely to be unsuccessful in dissuading Vicki from seeking amputation, Dr. Stayer believes she must try this first.[2]

After 9 months of psychotherapy and medication for anxiety and depression, Vicki's intense desire for amputation has not altered. If anything, the desire has increased. It has become more intense and is beginning to affect Vicki's daily activities.

Vicki returns to Dr. Stayer and pleads with her to perform the operation. Dr. Stayer is faced with a very difficult choice. Amputation is not a difficult or complicated medical procedure. Dr. Stayer has performed many amputations i.e., after an automobile accident, the remove a cancerous limb, or one with gangrene. But Vicki's case is different. She is in good health. Her left hand does not need to be amputated for any medical reason. Doing so will, in a sense, cripple Vicki. This is not what medical care is supposed to be all about.

---

[1] For a good overview for the layman see Carl Elliott, "A New Way to be Mad.", *The Atlantic*. (December: 2000); also see M.B. First, "Desire for Amputation of a Limb" *Psychological Medicine*. 34(2005): 1–10.

[2] It is well known that any form of psychotherapy is ineffective for Body Integrity Identity Disorder. It may even increase the desire for amputation. See Katharina Kroger, et al. "Effects of Psychotherapy on Patients Suffering from Body Integrity Identity Disorder" *American Journal of Applied Psychology*.3(2014): 110–115; D. Neff and E. Kasten, "Body Integrity Identity Disorder, what do Health Care Professionals Know." *European Journal of Counseling Psychology*. (2010): 16–30. Drug therapy has also proven ineffective. M.B. First, "Desire for Amputation of a Limb: Paraphilia, Psychosis, or a new type of Identity Disorder." *Psychological Medicine*. 35(2005): 919–928.

Yet talking to colleagues and studying relevant literature has shown Dr. Stayer the possible serious results of not doing the operation. Patients such as Vicki who are refused surgery frequently try to amputate the limb themselves. They use knives or saws, and they have no anesthetic and little sterile procedure.[3]

Such self-amputation can result in very serious adverse consequences. In other cases, patients have intentionally injured themselves so that emergency amputation is necessary. However, if they are not near a health care center or they injure themselves more seriously than they intended, worse results may ensue.

The etiology of this disorder is in dispute. Is it neurological or psychological? The current weight of the evidence seems to favor a neurological basis, but this remains in dispute.[4] It is known that most persons with this disorder are male and that 75% of those seeking amputation want the left and not the right hand amputated.[5] Those suffering from this problem are generally physically and psychologically healthy and they do not seek treatment for any illness. A significant number try to self-amputate, which frequently results in a surgeon finishing the job.

Mark Willis

Mark Willis is a 40-year-old, African American owner of a well-regarded house painting business in a suburb of a large city. He is happily married with two daughters and a son. For 2 days he has not been able to keep any food down and his abdomen is very distended. He vomits every few hours and must be near a toilet all the time.

His wife, Denise, drives him to the emergency room of a nearby hospital, where he is quickly diagnosed with an intestinal blockage. An IV for fluids and a nasogastric tube are quickly inserted in his arm and down his esophagus into his stomach. He is referred to Dr. Karen Rogers, the on call surgeon, who comes to see him immediately. Dr. Rogers informs Mark of the blockage and tells him that two likely causes are a tumor or a blockage of unknown origin. If it is not cancer, it may indicate Crohn's Disease. The only treatment right now is surgery to remove the blockage The surgery is not difficult. She had performed over 150 such surgeries with an almost 100 percent success rate. She asked Mark for his consent for surgery and for

---

[3] D. Bang, et al., "Aptomenophilia a Neurological Disorder", *Cognitive Neuroscience and Neuropsychology.* 19(2008): 1305–1306; P.D. McGoech, et al. "Aptomenophilia: The Neurological Basis of a Psychological disorder" *Nature Proceedings.* (2009): 1–5.

[4] H.M De Lisser, et al. "The Air Got to It: Exploring a belief About Surgery for Lung Cancer." *Journal of the National Medical Association* 101(2009): 765–771. M. George and M.L. Margolis, "Race and Lung Cancer Surgery: A Qualitative Analysis of Relevant Beliefs." *Oncology Nursing Forum* 37(2010): 740–748.

[5] J. Gregg and R.H. Curry, "Explanatory Models for Cancer among African American Women at Two Atlanta Neighborhood Health Centers: Implications For a Health Screening Program." *Social Science and Medicine.* 39(1994): 519–526.

his consent, if it was cancerous, to cut out all of it she could. and then refer Mark to an oncologist for further evaluation and follow-up.

Mr. Willis refused surgery. He was firmly convinced that if the tumor got air on it, the tumor would spread rapidly and kill him. Even if the tumor was not now cancerous, if air got on it, the result would be fatal.

A review of the literature shows Dr. Rogers that many persons have this patently false belief, or a closely related belief about the fatal effects of sunlight on a tumor. Such beliefs as these are not isolated or uncommon. In one study of women a significant majority of those studied believed that almost all cancer treatments did more harm than good. But the most negative beliefs were for "cutting" on a tumor.[5] In a large, multi-center study on lung cancer surgery, more than one third of the patients believed that air on a tumor would be fatal.[6] It seems that this belief is more common among Latino and African American populations. However, not enough research has been done to confirm this finding or to explore the causes for it.[7]

Dr. Rogers asks the hospital psychologist to talk to Mark to see if his belief can be altered and to see if he is competent to consent to or refuse this course of treatment. The psychologist reports that Mr. Willis' mind is firmly made up. Further, he reports that Mr. Willis does not give evidence of a neurological or psychological problem that would render him incompetent to refuse medical care.

However, the psychologist knows that given the ease with which persons can be found incompetent in court, Mr. Willis could probably be found incompetent.[8] This is especially the case since his wife strongly disagrees with his decision and would not contest a finding that he is incompetent. If he were found incompetent, she could easily make the decision for surgery.

Dr. Rogers is faced with a difficult decision. The blockage is well localized. If it is cancer it appears to be in an early stage. With surgery and chemotherapy, the success rate for treatment is over 90%.

---

[6] M.L. Margolis, et al. "Racial Differences Pertaining to Beliefs About Lung Cancer Surgery", *Annals of Internal Medicine*. 139(2003): 558–563.

[7] D.L. Lannin, et al. "Impacting Cultural Attitudes in African American Women to Decrease Breast Cancer Mortality," *American Journal of Surgery*. 184(2002): 418–423; C.M. Masi and S. Gehlert, "Perceptions of Breast Cancer Treatment Among African American women and Men,": *Journal of General Medicine*. 24(2008): 408–414; M.E. Fernandez, et al. "Colorectal Cancer Screening Among Latinos from U.S. Cities along the Texas–Mexico Border," *Cancer Causes and Control*. 19(2008): 195–206.

[8] see Paul Applebaum, "Assessment of Patients Competence to Consent to Treatment" *New England Journal of Medicine*. 357(2007): 1834–1840; J. Berg et.al, "Constructing: Formulating Standards or Legal Competence to Make Medical Decisions," *Rutgers Law Review* (1996): 345–396; T. Grisso and P. Applebaum, *Assessing Competence to Consent to Medical Care*. (New York: Oxford University Press, 1998). The varying standards reminds one of an incident years ago about televised boxing. The producer asked the boxing expert "where is this boxer ranked?" The response: "where do you want him ranked?" "There are so many different rating associations that he can be ranked almost anywhere." For an example see D. Marson, et al. "Assessing the Competency of Patients with Alzheimer's Disease Under Different Legal Standards." *Archives of Neurology*. 52(1995): 949–959.

The surgery is not difficult. She has performed many. She also knows that, with the strong support of his family, a finding that Mr. Willis is incompetent would not be difficult. She knows what she could do. But should she? The patient has firmly refused surgery. The finding of incompetency, while probably easy to obtain, is almost certainly a sham. The alternative, if it is cancer, though, is a slow and painful death, leaving his family bereft.

Ken Tidwell

Ken Tidwell is a 41-year-old white male with a long-standing diagnosis of schizophrenia. He lives on his own in a small apartment and spends his days in a program operated by the local Veterans Administration hospital. The program is housed in a renovated building right behind the hospital. The people being cared for here all receive VA benefits and Social Security disability payments. The people coming here can watch television, nap, play games, read, etc. They all have lunch every day.

The program is directed by a psychologist and a social worker. The social worker checks on the living arrangements of the people every week. A psychiatrist meets with each person every 2 weeks, to review their medication. For emergencies the hospital is less than a 100 yards away.

One morning the nurse observes that Ken seems to be sick. His abdomen is distended, and he vomits frequently. The psychologist accompanies Ken to the emergency room, where he is evaluated. A nasogastric tube is inserted in his esophagus to relieve the pressure on his stomach, and he is given a CAT scan that confirms the presence of an intestinal obstruction. The judgment of the surgeon, Dr. Dave Williams, and the gastroenterologist is that Ken requires surgery to relieve the blockage. It is about 9 am. Dr. Williams believes that he must operate by about 3 pm. The surgeon has performed over 200 such operations. He assures Ken that the operation is not difficult and is necessary to prevent a much more serious outcome that might threaten Ken's life.

Ken consistently refuses surgery with the same statement: "It is not time yet". His refusal is not obviously a sign of mental illness as it would be if he claimed that aliens were coming to cure him or that voices were telling him to refuse surgery.

The choice he is making may be irrational. But is he incompetent? The operation is not difficult and has a nearly 100% success rate. With his long-term diagnosis of schizophrenia, it would not be difficult to have Ken declared incompetent by a court. Someone else would then have to make the decision, a decision that would certainly be for surgery.

Dr. Williams is faced with a difficult decision. If he gets an emergency court order for surgery, what will be the long-term result? Will Ken become suspicious of all health care and abandon his outpatient care that has been very helpful for him? If Dr. Williams does not operate Ken could die or have his health seriously compromised.

Dr. Williams knows what he can do. But should he?

Linda Janko

Linda Janko is a 17-year-old young woman who is brought to the emergency room after a serious automobile accident. Examination in the emergency room shows that Linda has severe internal bleeding, a head contusion, and a fractured left femur. The femur is stabilized, and she is prepared for surgery to stop the bleeding. Without surgery Linda will almost certainly die within the hour. Surgery has a high likelihood of saving her life.

Her older sister, Jodi, was not injured in the crash. Jodi asks the surgeon, Dr. Adam Masley if the operation will involve blood transfusions. Dr. Masley said that with Linda's internal bleeding it would have to. No responsible surgeon would operate without transfusions, if needed. Then, Jodi states firmly that, as the only available "next of kin", she refuses blood transfusions, and that Linda would if she could. Jodi says that they are Jehovah's Witnesses. They have made a commitment to refuse blood transfusions based on what they believed God has revealed in the Bible.[9]

Dr. Masley is himself a deeply religious Catholic, so he respects their faith while not agreeing with their particular reading of scripture. To convince him of their sincerity Jodi shows him material published by the Watchtower Society in her sister's purse.[10]

Dr. Masley knows that some Jehovah's Witnesses will reluctantly accept transfusions if the blood is "forced" on them in an operation and the person was unable to refuse. He does not know if this "escape clause" will be acceptable here.[11]

The doctor knows that without an operation Linda will almost certainly die soon. The operation is very likely to save her life. He knows what he can do. But should he? In what sense is Linda's choice essentially different than the saints in his own Catholic Church, who chose to die for a good greater than life itself?

In the previous chapter we examined what I have called "epistemic uncertainty" in medicine. In those situations the doctor knows what he should do or what it is desirable to do. But the doctor is profoundly uncertain about whether he is able to do what it is desirable to do.

---

[9] The central text for Jehovah's Witnesses' is Leviticus 17:10–12 "Any Israelite or any alien living among them who eats any blood, I will set my face against that person who eats blood and will cut him off from his people, for the life of a creature is in the blood and I have given it to you atonement for yourselves on the alter. It is the blood that makes atonement. For ones' life. Therefore, I say to the Israelite none of you may eat blood."

[10] For a statement of the official doctrine see *Keep Yourself in God's Love*. (Watchtower Bible and Tract Society, 2008); Not all Jehovah's Witnesses practice this belief. In studies, between 10 and 20 percent of Jehovah's Witnesses do not agree: L.J. Findley and P.M. Redstone, "Blood Transfusion in Adult Jehovah's Witnesses" *Archives of Internal Medicine*. 142(1982):606–607; K. Benson, "Refusal of Transfusions by Jehovah's Witnesses" *Cancer Control Journal* 2(1995): 178–183.

[11] Lee Elder, "Why Some Jehovah's Witnesses Accept Blood and Reject Official Blood Policy," *Journal of Medical Ethics*. 26(2000): 375–380; also see Kurt Hartmann and Bryan Lang, "Exceptions to Informed Consent in Emergency Medicine" *Hospital Physician* 35(1999): 53–55.

II Equus

The cases above represent a different, and probably more common, form of uncertainty in medicine. I shall call this "moral uncertainty". In these cases, the doctor is confident about what he can do but is profoundly uncertain about whether she should do it.

Removing an intestinal blockage or amputating a hand are not difficult medical procedures. They are almost certain to be successful. But should a doctor dedicated to the health of the whole person maim, i.e., deform, the whole person or let the person die because of a patently false belief about the spread of tumors?

Are the alternatives any better? Should the doctor allow, by omission, the patient's health to be worse off by not professionally amputating her hand and forcing her to attempt self-amputation? Should the doctor let the young woman die for her faith like the martyrs his own faith celebrate? Might this patient accept a blood transfusion that she had no "control" over, such as during an operation when she is under anesthesia?

II Equus

The problem that these four cases illuminate is wonderfully described with a deeply religious shadow in Peter Shafer's 1975 Tony Award winning play and subsequent movie, *Equus*.[12]

The story of the play is, as follows. An adolescent English boy, Alan Strange has blinded a stable full of horses with a knife. A magistrate, Heather, has come to see her psychiatrist friend, Martin Dysart, to see if he will "treat" Alan to find out the background to this horrible deed. Further, she wants Martin to "fix" Alan so he will not do something like this again. Religious faith, it turns out, is at the heart of the problem for both Alan and Martin.

Alan grew up in a religiously divided household. His father, Frank, is a convinced atheist. Frank is not a quiet unbeliever. He is, rather, an outspoken and hostile atheist. As Frank tells Martin: "well look at it yourself. A boy spends night after night having this stuff read into him…bloody religion, it's our only real problem in this house, but its insufferable. I don't mind admitting it."[13]

Alan's mother, Dora, is deeply Christian in an evangelical/fundamentalist manner. Alan found a picture of Christ on his way to Calvary being whipped by Roman soldiers. Alan loved the picture and hung it over his bed. This attraction to it greatly pleased his mother.[14]

Frank hated it, as he did anything religious. In Dora's words: "He stood it for a while. But one day we got into one of our tiffs about religion and he went straight

---

[12] Peter Shaffer, *Equus*. (New York: Avon Books, 1975).
[13] Ibid. p. 39.
[14] Ibid. p. 51.

upstairs tore it off the wall and threw it in the dustbin."[15] Alan cried for days until he replaced the picture with one of a majestic horse.

To satisfy his religious hunger Alan has created another faith. He chants at night to an equine genealogy while whipping himself with a coat hanger, e.g., "prankus begat flankus, flankus begat spankus, spankus begat spunkus the great, leckwas begat neckwas, neckwas begat fleckwas and he said Behold I give you Equus my only begotten Son"[16]

Alan has fashioned his own religion patterned after the faith of his mother, with a horse, Equus, in place of Christ. It may be a warped faith and Christians will certainly regard it as false. But it is a faith, a belief in a higher power, that gives meaning to Alan's life.

Eventually Dysart uncovers the "why" of Alan's awful deed. He has met a girl, Jill. They start seeing each other. One night Alan and Jill have intercourse in the stable where Alan works. This is something that his mother had always told him is deeply wrong. Yet he has done this in the presence of the living symbols of his god. Thus, they must be blinded so they cannot see him anymore.[17]

Having finally uncovered the core of Alan's story and the reason for his horrible deed, Martin Dysart is faced with a terrible dilemma. As a psychiatric professional Dysart believes that he can "cure" Alan of his "warped" and destructive faith. In a manner, he can "normalize" Alan. This should be enough. But it is not.

Martin Dysart is a troubled soul. He is in a loveless marriage to a professional woman for whom he feels nothing. His wife, though highly educated, prefers the regular, the ordinary, the routine. Martin desperately wants more. As he tells Hester, "Do you know what it is like for two people to live in the same house as if they were in different parts of the world? She's always in some dreary kirk of her own inheriting. And I in some Doric temple, clouds tearing through the pillars, eagles bearing prophecies out of the sky".[18]

Martin wants the passionate relation to the transcendent, to what William James called the "more".[19] This "more" he does not have and does not know. He only knows that this is the object of his deepest desire and that he lacks it. He imagines, though, that it was much more to be found in ancient Greece. Dysart wants what Christians know as reverence or awe in the face of the transcendent. His most passionate desire is to be pierced with the flaming sword of love as St. Teresa of Avila said she was. A sword thrust by an angel. On the other hand, his wife, he coldly remarks, is "utterly worshipless". She cannot even recognize what Martin

---

[15] Ibid. p. 52.
[16] Ibid. p. 5.
[17] Ibid. pp. 113–120.
[18] Ibid. p. 71.
[19] The central text here is William James, *The Varieties of Religious Experience*. (New York: Penguin Library, 1982). These Gifford Lectures were given in 1901–2.

desperately desires. If she were pierced like St. Teresa, she would think herself mentally ill or physically sick.[20]

Martin Dysart's dilemma is both personal and professional. Alan's "faith", his connection to the transcendent, is, of course, abnormal. Almost certainly, his "faith" makes it difficult for Alan to hold a "normal" job and to lead an "ordinary" life. Yet it is this connection to a "more" that is not ordinary. As Dysart says: "The normal is the good smile on a child's eyes all right. It is also the dead stare on a million adults."[21] Alan's worship led him to do terrible things. But, Dysart says, "Without worship, you shrink. It's as brutal as that."

However, twisted Alan's specific "more" may be at least he has and feels a connection to a power beyond himself. Martin wants desperately what Alan has. What Alan has, however, leads into a horrific act. What now?

Should Martin sacrifice Alan's "more" on the altar of normality?

> Martin: "Can you think of anything worse one can do to anybody than take away? their worship?"
> Hester: "Worship isn't destructive Martin. I know that.
> Martin: "I don't. I only know that it's the core of his life. What else has he got?"[22]

For Martin, what gives Alan's life whatever meaning it has is Alan's "more" with his god, Equus. Without that, he has nothing. Martin knows what he can do. He knows what society expects him to do. What then? "He'll be delivered from madness. What then…do you think feelings like his can be simply re-attached like plasters stuck on to other objects we select? Look at him. My desire might be to make this boy an ardent husband, a caring citizen, a worshiper of an abstract and unifying God. My achievement, however, is more likely to make a ghost."[23]

For Christians what Dysart lacks is that passionate connection to God that is the gift of the Holy Spirit. Alan may have found a problematic spirit and what that connection led him to do is certainly terrible. But should his sense of the transcendent, the passion that gives his life meaning, be destroyed? Dysart's question remains haunting. Is there anything worse than destroying another person's faith?

Martin Dysart's dilemma is essentially the same as the doctors in the cases of Vicki, Mark, Ken, and Linda. Dysart and the others must choose a path. But each choice, each path, is imperfect. Should Dr. Stayer refuse Vicki's request for amputation? This refusal, however, might lead Vicki to attempt self-amputation with tragic results. Does Mark's patently false belief about cancer render him "incompetent" and give Dr. Rogers a way of doing surgery against his wishes? If the fundamental moral goal of medicine is *primum non nocere,* i.e. do no harm, is it not harm to let Mark die? In what sense is Linda's choice to die for her faith different than St. Stephen's death for preaching Christ to the Jerusalem authorities?

---

[20] St. Teresa of Avila *The Life of St. Teresa of Avila.* ed. Benedict Zimmerman. trans. David Lewis. (Gastonia, N.C.: Tan Books 1997).

[21] Equus. p. 74.

[22] Ibid. p. 93. St.

[23] Ibid. p. 123.

To act in the quandary he faces, both personally and professionally, Martin Dysart needs, more than he realizes, the very thing he lacks. Whichever way he turns, both personally and, professionally, with Alan, he must hope that good will come from his choice. He must hope that Alan will not become a ghost or a cypher working on an assembly line with little passion. To "cure" Alan, to remove the destructive spirit he has found, Dysart must hope that Alan will not end up as one of those millions of adults "with a dead stare"

Martin Dysart knows what he lacks, both professionally and personally. Like Socrates, he knows that he does not know. "Essentially, I cannot know what I do—yet I do essential, irreversible things. I stand in the dark, with a pick in my hands striking at heads."[24]

His humility in the face of the dark unknowing of his life and his profession reminds us immediately of St. Paul's words, that now we only see "through a glass darkly". In the words of St. John of the Cross, Martin is truly facing the "dark night of the soul". What Martin needs "more desperately than my children need me, a way of seeing in the dark". St. Paul's conclusion is what Martin does not grasp. "Now I know in part, then I shall know fully". If Martin has no way of grounding his hope in the "more", of being touched by the Holy Spirit, then his hope is no more than guesswork. His hope is in vain.

III Examing the Cases

The four cases we started with are deliberately chosen. Three are real, but appropriately made anonymous. Only the case of Vicki is fictitious but rooted in a real medical problem. The others are known to me, personally from my years teaching in a medical school.

Vicki's case involves the patient pleading with the doctor to do something positive to maim or deform a perfectly healthy person. The other three involve patient requests not to do something, to refrain from acting in ways the doctor believes is best.

The reasons that Mark, Ken and Linda do not want a medical intervention differ. Mark offers a reason based on a patently false belief about cancer. Ken offers no reason. Ken's lack of consent is stated calmly and, so far as an outsider can tell, not based on any obviously false belief, e.g., "aliens are coming to cure me". Linda offers a religious reason that those of no religion, another religion, or another Christian religion will reject. But she does not. Catholics will reject her specific faith, but their veneration of saints who willingly sacrificed their lives for a good higher than life is also regarded by outsiders, especially unbelievers, as unpersuasive, bizarre, or wrong.

---

[24] Ibid. p. 125.

III Examining the Cases

Of the four Vicki's case is, perhaps, the easiest to resolve. She is asking the doctor to positively harm her, to destroy the wholeness of body and soul that is the person, Vicki. Medicine's telos is to preserve, as much possible, the health of the person. Vicki is asking, even begging to be made less whole, less able.

Dr. Stayer cannot avoid considering the consequences of her refusal of her patient's plea. Vicki may search for another doctor. She may become more deeply depressed to the point that her daily life is seriously compromised. She may try to self-amputate, leading to much worse results for her physical health.

However, these remain possibilities, perhaps even probabilities, not certainties. They must be balanced against the operation which will render her less whole. For Vicki the operation will be a success if it permanently deforms her.

Yet, Dr. Stayer's refusal must be rooted not in certainty but hope. She must hope that Vicki's depression and anxiety do not deepen to an unbearable level, perhaps leading to a potentially fatal result. She must also hope that Vicki does not try to self-amputate with much worse results of pain, blood loss, and infection.

Though Vicki may see her situation as hopeless without an operation, Dr. Stayer must hope that the possibly grave results will not result. Where Vicki has little hope without harm, Dr. Stayer must act on a hope that is not essentially in vain. This is the hope that good will triumph over evil.

Linda's case is both harder in some ways and easier in others. The most difficult question cannot be answered with any certainty. What does Linda want? Her sister has a definite view. Linda would, if she could decide for herself, refuse surgery and die for her faith. It appears that this is what her sister, Jodi, would do. But what about Linda?

More information might help, e.g., information from more family and friends, or something in writing from Linda. Dr. Masley, however, cannot wait for such information. He must act now.

The easier part is that Linda's choice, if we presume that refusing blood is a choice that she would make, is not essentially different than choices made by committed believers in many faiths, especially Catholic saints who have been murdered for their faith. Dr. Masley may not share the specific faith that Linda and her sister have. He may find that the reading of the Bible by Jehovah's Witnesses wrong. But is the willingness to die for their faith any different than the willingness of St. Teresa de Benedicta of the Cross (Edith Stein) or St. Maximillian Kobe to die for theirs?

Yet Dr. Masley also must act in hope. He must hope that Jodi's choice is one that Linda would make if she were able too. He cannot know this. He must hope that Jodi's "choice" is essentially Linda's. He must also hope that for Linda there is a future beyond this moment where good will triumph over Linda's temporal death.

Dr. Masley must "hope against hope" that Linda can, in some manner, "look" as St. Stephen did, "and see heaven open and the Son of Man standing at the right hand of God". Dr. Masley must hope that, even when temporal realities appear grave and possibly hopeless, good will come out of a dire situation.

Mark is not incompetent. Any such finding by a court would be a sham. His belief about cancer is wrong, some might say it is absurd. Yet if we grant his belief, then his conclusion to refuse surgery is perfectly rational. Actually, this is an excellent example of the difference between truth and validity. His conclusion to refuse surgery is certainly valid if the starting point is accepted. But the argument does not lead to truth because the starting point is false.

Mark, as a person, is more than one false belief or many false beliefs. Mark is also a father, husband, homeowner, employer, churchgoer, and many other things. His business is well regarded. He is a loving husband, a kind father, a good employer. He sings in his church choir. Mark is more than a set of beliefs, no matter how false they may be.

To think of Mark as incompetent is to ignore Mark the person. It is to treat Mark as a means to an end, not an end in himself. Certainly Dr. Rogers and Mark's family and friends should try to persuade him to have the surgery. But coercing him, seems to treat Mark as less than a person and more as an object. To treat Mark as incompetent is to treat him as less than a person. Dr. Rogers and Mark's family must act out respect for Mark as a whole person. But they must also hope that, even in this difficult situation, good will triumph over the forces of darkness.

Respecting Mark as a person does not make the decision easier. If the blockage does not resolve itself soon Mark cannot be kept alive indefinitely with a nasogastric tube. Even if the blockage does resolve itself, cancer may still be present and without a biopsy Dr. Rogers will not know. Mark may die a slow and agonizing death. Dr. Rogers must hope that respecting Mark as a person will not entirely destroy Mark as a physical being.

Ken may be more easily found incompetent. He has a well established diagnosis of chronic schizophrenia which is controlled with medication. The medication helps with the symptoms, but it does not alter the underlying cognitive disability.

However, in refusing surgery Ken does not offer a bizarre or factually incorrect reason. He does not refer to aliens, voices, or psychic forces. Unlike Mark he does not offer a reason based on a factually incorrect belief. He offers no reason at all. His choice is one that few would make. His refusal may lead to very bad results for Ken's health. However, does Ken's refusal that seems "irrational" offer good grounds to find Ken as a person incompetent to refuse surgery such that Ken can be operated on over his objection. Ken is a person, not an object. If medicine' first rule is, "do no harm" is it not harm to treat Ken as an object, not a person.

To respect Ken's refusal Dr. Williams must act in hope. First, he can hope that Ken's blockage will relieve itself. Over 90% of such blockages do when the pressure is relieved with a nasogastric tube. But if it does not, hope remains at the center of Dr. Williams honoring Ken's refusal. If Dr. Williams thought only that horrible results would ensue from Ken's refusal, then he might feel compelled to act. But he cannot know this anymore than he can be sure about Ken's competency.

A finding that Ken is incompetent would ultimately have to rest on the seemingly irrational choice he is making. But such a move confuses competency with normality, i.e., the incompetent person will not make abnormal choices. Such a conclusion, however, leads to results in the cases of Linda and Mark that fail to respect them as persons.

Whichever choice Dr. Williams makes, he must hope that his choice and Ken's will lead to a conclusion he cannot now foresee. A hope that good triumphs over evil.

IV

The Psalmist writes that "You are my Hope, O Lord God, You are My Confidence". In each of the cases discussed above the doctor must act or refuse to act for what she believes are good and sufficient reasons. That is, he must act rightly and with confidence. But the doctor also must hope that the worst results will not follow from the decision he or she makes. This hope relies on a power that the psalmist calls "Lord God". Even physicians who are personally non-religious cannot act if they are paralyzed by fear of the unknown. Hope, not fear, gives confidence in the face of uncertainty.

In our first chapter we looked at hope through the lens of the great physician/moralists of the past Percival, Holmes, Kubler-Ross and Cabot. In Percival's words the physician must be a "minister of hope" to the sick and dying. As I argued there this idea is surely true. The doctor must not only be a mere technician, a scientific expert that treats the patient as an object not a human person. The person is far more than an object to be worked on with empirical skill as if he, the doctor, is carving a piece of wood or is equivalent to an auto mechanic or a computer programmer.

Yet, even as the physician is a minister of hope, she too must have hope, even in the darkest hour. Even when she cannot see clearly the road ahead, she must act with a hope that her patient will find a peace and a goodness that both he and her may not fully know.

Even those who have been given a witness of the Holy Spirit that few will ever attain recognize how little they actually know. As St. Paul writes "For now we see in a mirror darkly, but then face to face; now I know in part; but then I will know fully, just as I also have been fully known" I Corinthians 13: 12.

Whether the physician realizes it or not he is following the words of the Psalmist: "Reverence for the lord is the beginning of Wisdom".

Chapter 4
The Language of Hope

To better understand the concept of hope it will be helpful to examine what I will refer to as the "Logic of hope" or what we might think of as "the linguistics of hope" i.e. what our language of hope statement's reveal about nature of hope.

Consider these typical uses of the concept of hope:

I believe that Joe and Jane are going to get married.
I hope that Jane and Joe are going to get married.
Joe wants to go to medical school, so I hope that he does well on the MCAT (Medical College Admission Test)
Since she has studied hard and done well on practice tests, I believe that Jane will do well on the MCAT
Jane wants to go to a good law school, so I hope she does well on the LSAT (Law School Admission Test)
Joe is very intelligent and has studied hard. I believe he will do well on the LSAT
After seeing him at bars I believe that Sam is an alcoholic I hope Sam is not an alcoholic

These examples show two features of the language of hope that have been widely noted for a long time. But which are imprecise and are, therefore, often contested. The arguments are not over the general claims but over the details.

The first part of the language of hope is that it points to something that is uncertain.

To hold that one "knows" "that P," in a broad sense of "knowing" or that one believes that P implies that one has good grounds for one's belief e.g., Jane's native ability, Joe's scores on practice tests, Jane and Joe's love for each other.

The language of hope, however, requires no such good reasons for hoping that P. Jane's friends can hope that she does well on the MCAT without any knowledge about whether she had studied hard, how she has done on practice tests, or her native capacities. Joe and Jane's friends can hope that they will get married without any knowledge about how they feel about each other.

I

One can also hope that something is not true. One can hope that Lisa will not start smoking as her friends do or that Tom is not an alcoholic without any basis to believe whether there are any grounds for such a belief that "not P". I can hope that my friend does not have diabetes without any knowledge of his consistent blood sugar levels. Emily can hope that her husband does not have a broken leg from a fall off of a ladder, without any evidence whether he does or does not.

II

At the beginning of the Christian tradition Augustine provides concise discussion of hope in his *Enchiridion on Faith, Hope, and Love*. He makes 2 points. The first we have just seen.

Hope is not the same as belief. We can and do believe in things we should not hope for.

> What Christian, for example does not believe in punishment of the wicked? And yet such a one does not hope for it.[1]

In this sense, hope is grounded in uncertainty. For Augustine, we can have good grounds for believing Christ's death on the cross and his resurrection on Sunday morning. For Christians we can also believe or have faith in the salvation offered on the cross. I can only hope that I am among the saved who will be with God eternally.

For Augustine a second point is very crucial. A person can only hope for something that person regards as good. "Accordingly, faith may have for its object evil as well as good. For both good and evil are believed and the faith that believes them is not evil but good...But hope has for its object only what is good, only what is future, only what affects the man who entertains the hope. For these reasons, then, faith must be distinguished from hope not merely as a matter of verbal propriety but because they are essentially different"[2]

This second point, that what a person hopes for is regarded as good or desirable by that person is crucial. Yet stating this seemingly obvious point raises several complicated issues.

---

[1] Augustine, *The Enchiridion on Faith, Hope, and Love*. trans. Thomas Hobbs (Washington D.C: Regnery publishing, 1961): 9.
[2] Ibid.

If this point is granted, then can a person have wrong or false hope. If I hope for something bad or evil can that really be hope. Should it be thought of as "false hope"? Yet what makes it false as hope? Might it be better thought of as "disordered" or "distorted" hope? Should then "true hope" be understood as hoping for something actually good? Later in this chapter we will examine this problem closely.

III

Hope and Uncertainty

What has been called the "standard" or "orthodox" account of hope in recent years was given a reasonably precise statement by Robin Downie: "there are two criteria which are individually necessary and jointly sufficient for "hope that". The first is that the object of hope must be desirable by the hoper {the person who hopes} The second…is that the object of hope falls within the range of physical possibility, which includes the improbable."[3]

This standard account raises many questions. First, how uncertain must the event hoped for be? To hold that it must only be "unlikely" seems to place too stringent a requirement on hope. Another recent writer, J.P. Day offers a slightly more expansive version of hope when he writes that what a person hopes for must "have some degree of probability, however small".[4]

Other recent writers endorse this idea of likelihood or probability in even stronger terms. Phillip Pettit holds that "hope will consist in acting as if the desired prospect is going to obtain or has a good chance of obtaining".[5] Cheshire Calhoun writes that hope includes the "phenomenological idea of a determinate future whose content includes success".[6]

Downie, Day, and these other writers use the language of "probability" to understand the limits of hope. If it is probable or likely however, it doesn't appear to be an object of hope. One can only hope for what is "improbable" or "unlikely". But this seems too stringent. Downie, for example, holds that it is irrational to hope for an outcome that is "merely logically possible".[7] Other writers endorse a similar idea.

Consider this actual sports example, however. In 1951 in the National League baseball season the New York Giants were 13 games behind the Brooklyn Dodgers in late July with 50 games left to play. The hope of Giants fans that their team might

---

[3] Robin Downie, "Hope", *Philosophy and Phenomenological Research*. 24(1963): 248–251.

[4] J.P. Day, "Hope", *American Philosophical Quarterly*. 6(1969): 89–103.

[5] Phillip Pettit, "Hope and Its Place in Mind", *Annals of the American Academy of Political and Social Science*. 592(2004): 152–165.

[6] Cheshire Calhoun, *Doing Valuable Time: The Present, The Future, and Meaningful Living*. (London: Oxford University Press, 2020).

[7] Downie, op. cit. p. 249.

win the National League Pennant cannot be understood in terms of "unlikely" or "improbable". The Giants winning is not mathematically impossible but cannot be understood as only "unlikely". It does not, however, seem that the Giants' fans were completely irrational when they hoped that their team would win the National League title. Yet, in Downie's view it seems that this hoped for result was "merely logically possible".[8]

The position advanced in the standard account by Downie, Day and others was also presented in early modern thought by Hobbes and Descartes. In chapter six of *Leviathan* Hobbes discusses the cause of voluntary action in the passions (not reason). Fundamentally, Hobbes classifies all passions into groups. First are those that he calls "appetites" or "desires" for something the agent regards as good. Second are those results the agent hates or to which the agent has an aversion.

Whether Hobbes is right about this view of the causes of human action has been extensively debated. We shall not debate it here. In this context, however, he links hope with confidence. Confidence is identified by Hobbes as "consistent hope". This is a passion that is more than a one-time desire e.g.: "I hope it doesn't rain tomorrow so I can play golf" or "I hope I can win at the roulette table tonight".[9]

Essentially the same view is found in Descartes' *The Passions of the Soul*. He argues that hope is when "there is a good chance that something we desire will happen". Further, "when hope is extreme it changes its nature and becomes confidence".[10]

The standard account in its early version in Hobbes and Descartes or in the recent versions by Day and Downie raises many questions which are important to consider in this context, even if we must do so only briefly.

First, how uncertain must the event hoped for be? To hold that it must only be "unlikely" or in Day's language "in some degree probable" seems to place too stringent a requirement on hope. Surely it seems plausible to hope for an event that is more uncertain than merely "unlikely." The Giants' fans in 1951 are a case in point. Suppose a patient with breast cancer has a 15% chance of long-term survival. It is surely reasonable for that woman, her family, friends, and oncologist to hope for her long-term survival. Yet it certainly appears wrong to consider her survival as only "improbable" or "unlikely". Stabilizing Margaret Fuller's mood is not impossible for Dr. Henkson, but it is much more difficult than the language employed in the standard account seems to suggest.[11]

Once we have concluded that concepts like "improbable" place too stringent a limit on hope we must consider what the best alternative limit might be. There must be some limit. It makes no sense to say "I hope that aliens from vector nebula will come tomorrow and save Mark Willis' life". It makes no sense to say "I hope that

---

[8] The Online Book of Baseball.Com

[9] Thomas Hobbes, *Leviathan*. Ed. Richard Tuck. (London: Cambridge University Press, 1996).

[10] Rene Descartes, "The Passions of the Soul", in *The Philosophical Writings of Descartes*. vol. I eds. and trans. J. Cottingham, R Stoothhoff, D. Murdoch. (London: Cambridge University Press, 1985).

[11] Margaret Fuller's case.

my team can win the championship" when it is mathematically impossible for them to do so.

Perhaps the best alternative is to hold that the only lower limit to rational hope is to hold that what is hoped for is neither physically nor mathematically impossible. If a physician believes that there is only a 3% chance of this patient living longer than 6 months, it is not impossible for him or her to do so. From chapter two it is not impossible for Claire Darlington's life to be saved. If it were impossible, Dr. Gupta would not try to save her life.[12] It is possible that Dr. Frazier can remove all the cancer from Chuck's body and preserve his ability to have physical intimacy with Joan.[13]

However, making a judgment about what is possible or impossible cannot happen in a vacuum. These beliefs do not just appear *de novo*. They do not come from nowhere. Beliefs about what is possible are always nested in a background of other beliefs about: (1) oneself, (2) other persons, (3) the natural and social worlds, and (4) the transcendent or divine.

For example, suppose someone is opening a connivence store in a promising location that will sell gas, snacks, soda pop, beer, cigarettes, etc. One decision he or she must make is whether to install security cameras and if so, how many and where. This decision will be nested within a set of background beliefs about human nature in general and about the people who will patronize this particular store. This judgment might be different in a rural area than it would be in a major city.

Another example, more directly related to our topic involves the current idea of using genetic and other technologies to dramatically increase the human life span. Creating a life that is healthy at 150 or 175 years of age. One book in this extensive literature is by Terry Grossman m.d. and Ray Kurzweil (a computer science genius). The book is *Fantastic Voyage: How to Live Long Enough to Live Forever*. Whether their plan or any such plan is feasible cannot be assessed here. Suffice it to say that even if it were possible, it would take vast resources, perhaps billions of dollars to achieve.[14]

The rationality of such a pursuit is nested in a set of foundational beliefs about human nature and human destiny. If one believes that the life one has now is all the life one will have and that this life and the one in the future is a good life, it is hard to argue that it would be completely unreasonable for such a person to spend their resources in pursuing this goal.

On the other hand, if one believes that there will be a new life after death for individual persons, much better than this one with no pain, no worries and no death, a belief promoted by the great monotheistic religions of the west, it seems to be irrational for both individuals and societies to spend vast resources in this manner when basic resources like clean water are not available to millions of persons.

---

[12] Claire Darlington's case.

[13] Chuck's case.

[14] Terry Grossman m.d. and Ray Kurzweil, *Fantastic Voyage: How to Live Long Enough to Live Forever*. (New York: Plume, 2005).

In a recent essay Ariel Meirav has made this point in a slightly different manner. He asks us to consider two persons in the same situation of distress. On person despairs of a positive outcome in his/her situation. The other person hopes for a positive outcome. He argues that the difference between the persons in these cases is that the one who hopes believes in an "external factor" on which the positive outcome relies.[15]

The person who hopes does not know whether such a "factor" will intervene in this specific case. But this person believes that there is such a factor that might intervene in this case. The "external factor" may be Divine action, a breakthrough medical or pharmaceutical discovery, another person's arrival or many other unexpected persons or events. When a person hopes for divine action to intervene their hope based on a belief in an all-powerful, all-knowing and all-good God of the monotheistic religions of western civilizations: Judaism, Christianity, Islam. As an example, consider someone needing an organ transplant. They may have been on a transplant list for a long time without finding a matching donor. For this person the external factor might be a completely unknown and unexpected donor from a long way away.

Consider the material from Kubler-Ross. The patients she interviewed maintained their hope until their last days. They hoped for a dramatic cure, a new treatment, a new drug regimen, a new test that would show they were not fatally ill. Their hope was not grounded in a probability calculus. The idea of "unlikely" was not relevant to them. Downie's claim that persons should not hope for something that is merely "logically possible" was not a limit they recognized. They hoped, often passionately for an "external event" or "factor" to intervene. This intervention was not completely impossible (e.g. a body coming to life after having been dead for 5 days) but what they hoped for was extraordinarily unlikely.[16]

Perhaps, then, the lower limit to hope is to say that one cannot hope for what is physically impossible. Our physical bodies will not allow us to run a mile in under 2 minutes. If I am biologically a female, I cannot hope to be a biological male. I cannot hope that if I have XY chromosomes I can end up having XX chromosomes. I cannot hope that I can drive a gasoline powered car 1000 miles per hour. On the other hand, Kubler Ross' patients were hoping for an event that was not physically impossible but extremely rare. In this sense, the only events that are completely impossible are those that cannot physically come about, not those that are extremely rare. Only what we know is impossible cannot be a result we can hope for.

---

[15] Ariel Meirav, "The Nature of Hope", *Ratio*. 22(2008): 216–233.

[16] Tom Regan, *The Case for Animal Rights*. (Berkeley: University of California Press, 2004); David DeGrazia, *Animal Rights: A very Short Introduction*. (London: Oxford University Press, 2002); Cass Sunstein and Martha Nussbaum eds. *Animal Rights*. (London: Oxford University Press, 2005); Brittany Michaelson, *Voices for Animal Liberation*. (New York: Skyhorse, 2020).

IV

Hope and the Good

We shall now consider the second part of the standard account of hope which we have seen in Augustine's analysis and more recent work of Downie, Day, and others. This is the belief that what a person hopes for must, for that person, be considered good or desirable.

As a Christian theologian and philosopher Augustine believed that he knew for certain what the good is. The good is beliefs or activities that bring persons closer to God. Even basic things like food, water, and health care keep us alive and healthy so we can grow closer to God.

For those who are serious believers in any of the monotheistic religions this general concept of the ultimate human good and the goods that help us reach this final good is true. But to capture the language of hope in practice this idea of the good must be expanded.

Suppose a drunk driver has killed someone's wife or child in a terrible auto accident. This person has committed a grave moral wrong. In the wake of such a tragedy we often hear people say one of two things, (1) "I hope he gets what is coming to him" or (2) "I hope he gets what he deserves".

The first statement is a tautology. A person will always get "something" in the future, i.e., what is coming to them. But the second statement perfectly sensible, even if what I believe a person deserves is quite horrible, e.g., being burned at stake or starved to death.

No system of morality can plausibly justify either of these "punishments". Being burned at the stake, starved, or tortured are wrong in the strongest possible way. Hence, what does it mean to hope that someone receives one of these punishments? In my view the only plausible answer is that the person who hopes that someone receives one of these punishments believes that this result is good for the person being punished.

As a result, it seems that one can hope for a result that is morally wrong, even drastically wrong. But the person who hopes for such a result may not realize the moral standing of that for which he or she hopes. To hope, the person who hopes must believe that the result they hope for is actually good. The person who killed his wife as a drunk driver must get what he believes she deserves, even if what he hopes her punishment will be is morally wrong.

It seems, therefore, that there are three alternatives to connect hope with a concept of good or desirable. The first is to deny that hoping for something such a criminal being tortured is actually hope. Hitler hoping to eliminate every Jewish person in Europe is not actually hope. A school shooter who hopes to kill those who he believes bullied him at school is not actually hoping because he does not hope for something actually good.

In these and similar cases what is wanted can often be referred to as "vengeance" or "revenge" language that seems more negative than what is generally thought of as something to "hope" for. But this move seems like a word quibble that does not work.

If I actually hope for it, it must be something good
What I hope for is not good
Therefore, what appears to be hope, cannot be actual or true hope

This approach is purely stipulative and does not reflect our ordinary language of hope.

A second approach is relativist. On this account what I hope for must be good for me. If I hope for something happening to another person that seriously hurts that person, then, for me the result must be good.

I hope for some result in the future.
I can only hope for what I believe is a good result.
Hence, I must believe that this result is good.

To hold this view of hope, one must hold that moral relativism is correct. What I believe is good must be good for me. Moral relativism, however, has been shown to have several serious problems, which can be briefly noted here.

First, our moral language simply does not reflect complete moral relativism. On a wide range of issues people disagree about practical moral problems, both in general and in specific cases: abortion, capital punishment, war, affirmative action, the moral standing of animals, etc.

These disagreements are real and significant. As are disagreements about the best moral theory to employ in examining these questions. One point is often overlooked when examining these debates. Both sides or many sides of these debates believe that they are right. They are not relativists.

Consider, for example, the moral worth of non-human animals, what are often referred to as "charismatic mega fauna". Animal rights advocates do not say "I will not hunt, but if you want to that's fine". They think hunting is wrong for everyone. They do not say "I am a vegetarian, but if you like a steak dinner go ahead" The animal rights advocates believe that their view is right, and the views of deer hunters and meat eaters is wrong.[16]

A second example is capital punishment. Supporters believe that in some especially vicious cases capital punishment is right, for various reasons. Opponents do not say.

"I don't want it in my state, but if you want it in your state, that is alright". No, they believe that it is wrong always and everywhere.[17]

In a third example consider female circumcision. Feminists and others do not believe that this practice should be allowed in cultures where it is practiced and has been for millenia.

---

[17] Hugo Adam Bedau, ed. *The Death Penalty in America*. (London: Oxford University Press, 1997); Stuart Bonner, *The Death Penalty: An American History*. (Cambridge: Harvard University Press, 2002); Evan Mandary, *The Death Penalty in America*. (Burlington, MA: Jones and Bartlett, 2011).

Critics believe that the cultural relativist argument for allowing the practice to continue in some areas of the world is just wrong.[18]

In these and numerous other cases our general way of thinking and talking about morality does not support relativism. Of course, there are vigorous debates about moral issues, moral systems, and the grounding of morality in human existence, both personal and social. But all sides believe that there is a correct way of thinking about specific issues and the foundations of morality.

If the first alternative does not reflect the ordinary language of hope and the second alternative relies on a relativism that moral disagreement rejects, we should consider a third alternative.

This alternative rejects relativism and does not distort our common language of hope.

This view holds that what a person hopes for must be thought of as good or desirable by that person. But that person may be wrong. What he or she believes is good may not actually be good. Provisionally I shall call this hope for a result that is not actually good "disordered hope". What the person who hopes believes to be good is not actually good.

Hitler hoped to eliminate the Jewish people from Europe. For him is this was an ultimate good. But when others realized that for him this was a desirable goal and thought about it they knew that though he hoped for it, this goal was evil, not good. A man hopes to murder his ex-girlfriend's new boyfriend. For him this result is good. He desires this goal. Others believe that this result is wrong and his hope as disordered.

Hitler, Stalin, bank robbers, this ex-boyfriend and innumerable others do hope for what they believe is good. Hitler was not a relativist. He and others just noted are seriously wrong in many ways. But to say they do not actually hope is wrong. This third alternative captures these disordered hopes.

V

The two fictional physicians we have seen in Chaps. 2 and 3 represent powerfully the questions raised by language of hope. Bernard Rieux has no doubt about what the good is for himself and the people of Oran in this crisis: eliminate the plague that is destroying life in Oran.

Oran is dying both physically and psychologically. To end this misery and suffering is the overarching goal of all of his actions. Right now, this is the true good.

When Castel's "serum" is ready to test, Rieux has no hesitation in testing the "serum" on a young boy. Yet he has very little belief that this treatment will save the

---

[18] Rosemarie Skaine, *Female Genital Mutilation: Legal, Cultural and Medical Issues.* (Jefferson, N.C.: McFarland,2005); Martha Nussbaum, *Sex and Social Justice.* (London: Oxford University Press, 1999); Kandala Ngianga Bakwin and Paul Komba, *Female Genetal Mutilation.* (Berlin: Springer, 2018).

life of the boy. For Rieux this goal is not merely "improbable" or "unlikely". For Rieux success is not actually impossible as it would have been if the boy had been dead for days. But the standard language of hope reflected in the concepts of probability or likelihood does not reflect Rieux's situation.

Of course, Rieux and Castel would not act as they do if the situation were completely hopeless. But the hope of Rieux and Castel is so low in probability that it could be colloquially referred to as "hopeless". Yet they act anyway. They are, in Percival's language, "ministers of hope". Unlike actual ministers or like Father Paneloux who pray to a God whose ways they do not know and cannot understand, Rieux and Castel hope for a result that is almost impossible, unless the actual god of Percival and Paneloux intervenes with what would be an actual miracle.

Martin Dysart does not doubt that he can successfully "treat" Alan Strang. Given the uncertainties of psychiatric medicine he probably should have doubts. But he does not. He is confident that he can return Alan to a normal life. He can "normalize" Alan. But Dysart, both personally and professionally, questions whether the "normal" is the good. Admittedly, Alan's abnormality has led him to do a terrible thing. There can be no doubt about this moral judgment. Yet Martin Dysart raises the most profound question. Is the abnormal always bad or wrong.

Consider the great religious leaders of the past. Jesus rejected the pharisaic focus on minute rules and the Sadducees rejection of resurrection. Mohammed rejected the polytheism of Mecca in his day. The great Jewish prophets rejected the polytheism and henotheism of their era; Proclaiming instead, "our God is one God." Martin Luther King rejected the "normality" of the racism and segregation of his day, it was not good. It was evil.

So also do the great mystics in several traditions reject normality. Christians: St. Teresa of Avila, St. Hildegard of Bingen, St. John of the Cross. Islam: Al Shah. Ibn Arabi, Al Khutwa. Judaism: Kabbala, Zohar, Hasidism.

Dysart deeply questions whether what is thought to be normal, or routine is actually good. He wants a life touched or even transformed by the transcendent. For Dysart, what makes life worth living is not the normal. He wants what Alan has found, just not his version of it. He is afraid that the only way to successfully treat Alan is to turn him away from the transcendent. Dysart believes that he must numb Alan to what William James referred to as the "more". Alan must think only about the body, not about the soul.

To employ our previous discussion, Alan's hope is "disordered". Dysart believes that to "order" Alan's hope properly he must get Alan to stop hoping or thinking about the "more". Dysart himself desires this "more" but he does not know how to come to it or experience it.

Conclusion

The general language of hope is not problematic. Downie's view is broadly correct. We employ the language of hope when we are uncertain about a future event. Also, we do not hope for something we, the person who hopes, regards as bad or wrong. The person hopes for what he or she regards as good.

There are, however, two sorts of hope. The first is what we can refer to as temporal hopes: a better job, more education, a better house. In the instances we started this chapter with a good score for Jane on the MCAT, a good score for Joe on the LSAT, a good marriage for Joe and Jane.

The second sort of hope is what we can refer to as transcendent hopes. These is "hope for" that is not merely limited or temporal. This is hope for that must involve a case beyond the momentary or easily seen and understood. This hope relies on a power that can bring about a good that we can recognize as good but can only partially understand how it came about.

In the next two chapters we will carefully examine temporal and transcendent hopes

Chapter 5
Hope and Temporal Goods

When the Roman Empire became officially Christian in the fourth century a number of educated Romans thought that they could create a truly Christian civilization that governed by Christian principles, treated citizens with respect, and ruled virtuously with real justice. Though the Roman elite admitted that that heaven was still heaven, they seemed to aspire to a truly "City of God" on earth.[1]

These hopes were crushed when the Visigoths invaded Rome in 410. Many of the elite Romans fled to North Africa, where Augustine was able to hear and understand the story of their original hopes for a "heaven on earth" and how these aspirations were destroyed when what they regarded as an uncivilized, savage group destroyed what they regarded as the greatest city on earth.[2]

Hearing these stories moved Augustine to write one of his masterpieces the *City of God* in this massive work Augustine argues that there are two cities: an earthly city and a heavenly city. They can be regarded as the city of man and the city of God. What Augustine refers to in this work is two forms of human existence and two forms of human good. There is an earthly life in the earthly city. This city fosters and preserves earthly goods: the physical life of human beings, punishing criminals, setting out laws that citizens should follow to preserve peace, establishing rules for property, governance, and many other temporal goods.[3]

The second city is the heavenly city, the City of God. In this city all the evils, distresses, and sadness of life in the earthly city are no more. Human persons are eternally happy with no wants or needs. They are held in God's arms of love forever.

---

[1] Peter Brown, *Augustine of Hippo: A Biography*. 2nd ed. (Berkley: University of California Press, 2000): 285–312.

[2] Peter Heater, *The Fall of the Roman Empire*. (London: Oxford University Press, 2000).

[3] Augustine, *The City of God* trans. Henry Bettenson (London: Penguin, 1972). Also see James Weitzel, *Augustine's City of God: A Critical Guide* (*London*: Cambridge University Press, 2012).

This city will never collapse or be overrun by enemies, opponents, or forces of evil. This city embodies the true, complete, and final human good.[4]

These two cities embody the two fundamental human goods: the temporal goods of this world and the heavenly goods that are the end or telos of all our striving. In each case we have a general idea of the nature of the city and some idea of its organization, but we can only hope that we, as persons, are or can be citizens of such a city.

Here in this temporal world humans must hope that the actual city in which they live provides well the temporal goods necessary for life here: e.g., protection of life and property, laws that define crime, a fair system of investigation and punishment, dealing with persons fairly and justly. We can know what a good earthly city is like. We must hope that we can live in such a city.

We can also have some idea about the heavenly city and how human beings will be eternally happy and fulfilled in this city. What we must hope is that we will be citizens of this heavenly city. We cannot know this. We must hope for this result for ourselves, our families, those we know, and for everyone.

I Socialism and Temporal Hope

Those who seek a temporal good civilization are manifold in human history. The Israelites were fleeing from Egypt to a promised land one "flowing with milk and Honey". Abraham was led from "Ur of the Chaldees" to a promised land. The Puritans came to New England in the early seventeenth century to build a temporal perfect society, as did the Mormons who sought an earthly kingdom of God in the intermountain west in the middle of the nineteenth century.

All of these attempts were supposedly led by God to build a special community on earth whether small or large. These founders and followers tried to build an earthly community following a divine plan.

One of the greatest epic poems in western literature presents a powerful story of this struggle to create a good temporal civilization which the founder must hope that he and those he leads can found. This is Virgil's *Aeneid*, the story of Aeneas' journey and struggle to found Rome. Aeneas represents the losing side of the Trojan war. He leads a group of the "losers" on a long journey with detours along the way to found the great earthly civilization of Rome.[5]

His journey is not predetermined. His path is uncertain; some of the gods want him to succeed and some do not. Aeneas and those who follow him cannot know that they will succeed in establishing a good temporal civilization. Unlike the Israelites who claim to know that fleeing Egypt's slavery is led by God or the Mormons settling in the intermountain west, Aeneas and his followers are not

---

[4] *City of God.*
[5] Virgil, *The Aeneid* trans. Robert Fitzgerald. (New York: Random House, 1983).

following a divine plan or playing a part in a divine script. They must hope that their efforts can succeed.

None of these classical founders were thought at the time to have a predetermined result. Ulysses' years of returning from the Trojan war and the troubled journey he took was not predetermined either by fate or a divine source. Neither was Aeneas 'journey to found Rome pre-determined.[6] The gods intervened considerably in Aeneas' journey, but they did not predetermine a result. If the difficulties faced by Ulysses and Aeneas were predetermined by God, we would be led to consider what kind of God would deliberately cause those whose fate is in his or her hands to suffer so much.

Neither do the journeys of Moses and Abraham appear to be predetermined. Abraham is told that he will be shown a beautiful land where he and his offspring can flourish, not that they will. That is yet to be determined. Neither is Moses told that his journey with the Israelites out of Egypt is predetermined to succeed. Of course, in both cases, God intervenes frequently. Saving Abraham's cousin Lot from Sodom. Opening the Red Sea for the Israelites to pass through, ensuring that the Israelites have food and water in the desert. But in neither case is the result determined. Both Abraham and Moses must hope that for each of them and their followers good will come out of their journeys and struggles[7] Whether the earthly goods that they desire and a society of peace and plenty will result they cannot know. They must hope.

These examples from ancient literature and the Bible show that the achievement of a temporal good society must be rooted in a hope that good will triumph over evil. One could cite many other examples from ancient and medieval literature about the striving for a temporal good society in which humans can flourish with peace and security. All of these journeys are rooted in the hope that this good can be realized. We should also cite the American founders who pledged "their lives, their fortunes, and their sacred honor" on the hope that America could be a beacon to the rest of the world.

II

In modern times this vision of a good temporal society without tyranny or dictatorship and a place of security and justice has been powerfully promoted by socialist thinkers especially Marx, Engels, and their followers. In its early classical form, especially from Engels and less forcefully Marx, Marxism did not need the concept of hope because it was highly deterministic. The future communist utopia would be

---

[6] Efstraios Sarischoulis, "Fate, Free Will, and Narrative Concept in the Homeric Epics", *Mythos* 10(2016):81–115.

[7] Abraham is told that he will found a great earthly nation and that "all the people of the earth" will be blessed through him, *Genesis* 12; Moses' story in Exodus promised a land "flowing with milk and honey." *Exodus* 3:8.

realized. As we have seen, however, hope is a concept that is used when a result is not only desired but uncertain. The Marxist vision of a society with peace, security and human flourishing is highly desirable. But if the Marxist is certain that it will happen, he or she does not hope that this utopia will come to pass. They know that it will happen. It Is not hoped for; it is waited for. Achieving this utopia may take hard work and the journey may be long and difficult but the result is certain.

One can hope for the short-term success of a particular program as some, nineteenth-century radicals hoped for the success of the Paris Commune or the revolutions of 1848.[8] But this sort of Marxist did not need to hope for the ultimate coming forth of their utopia.

The most powerful statements of this Marxist economic determinism is from Engels short work *Socialism Utopian and Scientific* which is part of a larger work *Herr Eugen Duhring's Revolution in Science*. *Socialism Utopian and Scientific* is actually only a short pamphlet useful for popular distribution and can be easily read and understood by any literate person.[9]

In this work and the larger more complete statement in what is known as *Anti-Durhing Engels* is completely deterministic. The question of whether Marx himself was as deterministic as Engels is a matter of debate. But Marx did endorse the first edition of *Anti-Durhing* which was published while he was alive.

In his work, both *Anti-Durhing* and the shorter pamphlet, Engels explicitly criticizes what he refers to as a utopian version of socialism, a socialism that is optimistic and desirable but uncertain. Many of those who were in this group including, Durhing, Eduard Bernstein. and August Babel rejected determinism.[10] They thought that socialism was desirable. They aspired to a socialist society. However, they did not believe that it would surely come about. For example, Babel and Bernstein both served in legislatures in Germany, which would be irrational if socialism were going to come about. Thus, for these thinkers hope in an earthly utopia was important.

Engels strongly rejected this aspirational socialism. For Engels, Marx had discovered the laws of social and economic development as surely as Darwin had discovered the law of evolution in the biological world. Biologists can debate some of the details of evolution but to debate the general theory, for Engels, would be nonsense. Engels often compares Darwin's law of evolution with Marxist law of economic development. To debate either one is irrational. At Marx's gravesite

---

[8] Robert Tombs, *The Paris Commune*. (New York: Routledge, 2014); Alaister Horne, *The Fall of Paris: The Siege and the Commune*. (London: Picador, 2012); William Langer, *The Revolutions of 1848* (New York: Harper, 1971); Peter Steerns, *The Revolutionary Tide in Europe* (New York: W.W. Norton, 1974).

[9] Friedrich Engels, *Socialism: Utopian and Scientific* Available on line at www.Marxists.org. Friedrich Engels, Herr *Eugen Duhrings Revolution in Science* Available at Marxists.org

[10] Peter Gay, *The Dilemma of Democratic Socialism*. (New York: Columbia University Press, 1952); Manfred Steger, *The Quest for Evolutionary Socialism*. (London: Cambridge University Press, 1997); Gary Steenson, *Karl Kautsky: 1854–1938: Marxism in the Classical Years*. (Pittsburgh: University of Pittsburgh Press, 1978).

Engles pronounced just as "Darwin discovered the law of the development of organic nature, so Marx discovered the law of the development of human history."[11]

Finally, one of the most important students of Marxism writes of this turn to rigid determinism after the death of Marx: "the drift toward positivism and scientism accelerated after his death and formalized by Kautsky after Engles in his turn had left the field went from far beyond anything he can have envisioned in place of the original dialectical conception in which critical thought was validated by revolutionary action, there now appeared a cast-iron law from which the inevitability could be deduced with an almost certain mathematical certainty".[12] In this world there is no need to hope.

Whether Marx himself was fully and completely deterministic is a matter of scholarly debate that need not concern us here. Not all of those who considered themselves Marxist are deterministic. We have already noted some of the aspirational Marxists whom Engels strongly opposed.

III

In the recent post World War II period no Marxist thinker has done more to rehabilitate the open Marxism of the past than the German philosopher Ernst Bloch. His masterpiece *The Principle of Hope* is a powerful statement of a Marxism that is not deterministic. The title itself reflects this. As we have seen hope reflects a desire and an uncertainty. This aspirational Marxism lays out the power of hope in human life, the freedom and uncertainty in our pursuit of what we hope for, and the final "kingdom of God" on earth that Marxism can achieve.[13]

Bloch was born in 1885, 2 years after Marx's death. His parents were assimilated Jews. His father wanted him to study practical subjects, e.g. engineering. At a nearby library, however, Bloch read extensively in German philosophy especially Hegel and others of that period. He studied in Munich and Wurzburg. In Berlin he was part of a study group assembled by George Simmel He also studied with Max Weber, His dissertation was on the epistemology of Heinrich Reichart, an important neo-Kantian of the period.[14] It was published by the University of Wurzburg. In Heidelberg he began his lifelong friendship with Gorg Lukacs. Bloch taught Lukacs western philosophy and Lukas introduced Bloch to Dostoevsky, Kierkegaard, and German mysticism especially Hildegard of Bingen.[15]

---

[11] Friedrich Engels, *Speech at Marx's Gravesite 1883*. at Marxists.org

[12] George Lichtheim, *Marxism: A Historical and Critical Study*. (New York: Praeger, 1964):238.

[13] Ernst Bloch, *The Principle of Hope* trans. Neville Place, Stephen Place, Paul Knight 3 vols. (Cambridge: MIT Press, 1986). Hereafter PH.

[14] Sebastian Luft ed. *The Neo-Kantian Reader*. (New York: Routledge, 2015); R.G. Collingwood, *The Idea of History*. (London: Oxford University Press, 1946).

[15] Vincent Geoghegan, *Ernst Bloch*. (New York: Routledge, 1996); Arpad Kadarskay, *Georg Lukacs: Life, Thought, and Politics*. (London: Basil Blackwell, 1991); W. Jung, "The Early

In the 1920s he lived several places in Europe. When Hitler came to power he fled to Switzerland and several other places. Eventually he came to the United States where he lived from 1938 to 1949 most of this time he lived in Cambridge Massachusetts.[16] He was one of many secular Jewish leftists who fled from Europe in the wake of Hitler's rise to power e.g. Simone Weil, Theodore Adorno, Max Horkheimer, Herbert Marcuse, Eric Fromm. Though not a leftist Leo Strauss comes from this same milieu.

In the 1940s Bloch had high hopes of joining the Institute for Social Research which fled Germany and was attached to Columbia University. But the key leaders, especially Horkheimer and Adorno rejected him as being too communist, which is ironic because while he supported the Soviet Union at the time, his major work *Principle of Hope* is Marxist humanism at its best.

In 1948 he was appointed to succeed Gadamer at the University of Leipzig. During the 1950s his anti-Stalinist position got him repeatedly into conflict with the east German authorities. Finally, the building of the Berlin wall in 1961 caused him to move to West Germany and accept a position at the University of Tubingen.

Bloch did not come of age as a Marxist. It wasn't until his late 30s, in the 1920s, that he started to develop a self-conscious Marxism. The first edition of *The Spirit of Utopia* in 1923 does not really touch on Marx or Marxism. Neither does his fascination with radical religious figures Joachim of Fiore and Thomas Munzer. Joachim foretold the coming of an age of the spirit which was essentially a renewed and perfect earth governed by the Holy Spirit. Munzer tried to build a kingdom of God on earth in the 1520s.[17] What united these thinkers and others that Bloch was attracted to was their focus on a renewed human life on earth without wants, worries or greed. When he came to Marxism, it was as a Marxist different than the reigning dogmas of Engels, Kautsky, Lenin, and Stalin.[18]

This difference is seen first in the way in which he employs the concept of utopia in a manner almost the opposite of that employment by Engels and the supposedly standard form of Marxism. If Engels contrasts utopian visionary socialism with the true scientific Marxism, Bloch would certainly be in the utopian camp.

Aesthetic Theories of Bloch and Lukacs", *New German Critique*. 45(1988):41–54; E. Kardi, "Bloch et Lukacs dans le Cercle de Weber" in P. Furlan, A. Munster, N. Tertulian eds. *Réification et Utopia: Ernst Bloch et Gyorgy Lukacs Siècle*. (Arles: Acts Sud, 1986):69–87; Ivan Boldyrev, *Ernst Bloch and his Contemporaines: Locating Utopian Messianism*. (London: Bloomsbury Publishers, 2015).

[16] Geoghegan: 18–19.

[17] Bernard Whalen, *The Dominion of God: Christianity and Apocalypse in the Middle Ages*. (Cambridge: Harvard University Press, 2009); Norman Cohn, *The Pursuit of the Millennium Revolutionary Millenarians and Mystical Anarchists of the Middle Ages*. (London: Oxford, 1970); Werner Gould and Marjorie Reeves, *Joachim of Fiore and the Myth of the Eternal Evangel in the 19th and 20th Centuries*. (London: Oxford University Press, 2001); Tom Scott, *Thomas Muntzer: Theology and Revolution in the German Reformation*. (London: Macmillan, 1989).

[18] See the introduction to *PH* See also J.O. Daniel and T. Moylan eds. *Not Yet Reconsidering Ernst Bloch*. (London: Verso Books, 1997). M. Blechman, "Not Yet: Adorno and the Utopia of Consciousness," *Cultural Critique* 70(2008): 177–198.

III

The foundation of Bloch's masterpiece is the observation that hope for a better world and a better life for persons in this world is part of human nature. It has been so from the beginning of human existence and will always be so. Bloch's central concern for the future is the concept of "not yet". This stands between always or determinism and never, another form of hard negation. Both of these alternatives have no place for the concept of hope, since hope is grounded in uncertainty that each of these denies.[19]

Though not religious, Bloch's use of the concept of hope means that for him the earthly future of humankind is often not closed. The openness of the "not-yet" is seen at every stage of individual human life and in every civilization that strives for better existence on earth. Not a kingdom of God in the heavenly realm but a renewed and reformed civilization here in our world. Bloch's masterpiece has a deep connection to biblical religion. In a profound way he takes eschatological aspirations of biblical faith for a "city of god" and brings them to earth, as Prometheus brought fire to humanity.[20] We should also note that Bloch's study of hope as a "master concept" of human existence influenced the "theology of hope" movement among especially protestant theologians in the 1960s and 1970s.

The first section of the *Principle of Hope* is devoted to daydreams.[21] Of course, daydreams are often otherworldly and trivial. But their commonality and universality illustrate the pervasiveness of human beings dreaming about what they do not have and desire. That is, what they hope for: a new job, a better house, new friends, different climate to live in. From this fact, these daydreams illustrate the pervasiveness of human hope for something good in the future. From this beginning, human persons develop more extensive and deeper dreams.

These more extensive dreams can involve new civilizations or cities of wealth and power: e.g., El Dorado that many Spanish conquistadors tried to find or Atlantis, the legendary Island west of the Pillars of Hercules (Gibraltar) mentioned by Plato in his *Critias* and *Timaeus*.[22] More recent examples are dreams of humans colonizing other planets or using robots to perform our manual labor.[23] These sorts of dreams are for Bloch forward-looking not retrospective. The conquistadors searched for wealth in their day as did those who longed for Atlantis. The Europeans who

---

[19] *PH* 21–41; L. Weissberg, "Philosophy and the Fairy tale: Ernst Bloch as Narrator," *New German Critique*. 55(1992): 21–44 Ernst Bloch, "The Fairy Tale Moves on its Own in Time" in Ernst Bloch, *The Utopian Function of Art and Literature* .eds. and trans. Jack Zippes and Frank Mechlenberg (Cambridge, MA: MIT Press, 1988): 163–166.

[20] Pierre Vidal-Naquet *The Atlantis Story: A Short History of Plato's Myth*. (Exeter, U.K.: Exeter University Press); John Hemming, *The search for El-Dorado*. (New York: E.P.Dutton, 1979).

[21] Cameron Smith and Evan Davies *Emigrating Beyond Earth*. (New York: Springer, 2012); Joseph Fletcher, *The Ethics of Genetic Control*. (New York: Anchor Books, 1974); Hugo de Garis, *The Artilect Wars*. (New York: ETC Publishing, 2005).

[22] Angell Pearson, *Henri Bergson: An Introduction* (New York: Routledge, 2011).

[23] Jay Hetrick, "The Uses and Abuses of Bergson in Critical Theory," "*Cosmos and History: The Journal of Natural and Social Philosophy.*" 17(2021): 99–136.

followed Columbus and sailed west in the Atlantic Ocean hoped not only to find gold but also a passage to the orient and new lands to claim for their countries.

After arguing that these sorts of "not yet" dreams are a core part of human nature Bloch turns to showing how this "not yet" connects to our everyday world in an enormous number of ways. Bloch himself employs a limiting psychology of human drives, at this point, but his point is clear. Humans have a desire for what they do not have and believe that what they do not have, is good: power, wealth, a longer life, better health etc. Bloch regards reality as a process and that the future is open.

But the openness of the future is ultimately grounded in the present; this grounding of the "not yet" is in what is possible. Bloch knows we might and often do dream of what is not possible. Nightmares and literature are filled with such dreams. For example, the Emerald City of Oz, Alice's Wonderland, Don Quixote, Star Trek, or Star Wars "a long time ago in a galaxy far away". But these are dreams we cannot hope to be realized because they are not grounded in any reality.

This focus on what is actually possible is crucial in his dispute with his older somewhat contemporary Henri Bergson. He argued that Bergson's "creative evolution" was a grander version of wish fulfillment, "somewhere over the rainbow",[24] ungrounded in reality and oblivious to the contradiction of capitalism. The future is open, for Bergson, but it's openness is not grounded in the realities of both the present and human nature that does not change. Bloch's view is that Bergson's is an openness to the future that cannot be a true openness to transformative possibilities because its vision is framed by the bourgeois world of its era.[25]

The fundamental problem of creating what Bloch would recognize as a true utopia is to bring together human beings and nature, capitalists, and workers, rich and poor, freedom and necessity, past and present, men and women, young and old.

Bloch has analyzed extensively faulty claims of utopianism and faulty attempts to create an earthly utopia beginning with his early book on Thomas Munzer;[26] but a real utopia brings together the things that divide us. The present is grounded in the past but has grown beyond it. Capitalism divides people into social and economic classes. Capitalist leaders seek to dominate nature for material gain. Since socialism provides for everyone equally the desire for material gain will diminish and a balanced relation with nature and other people will result.

Unlike some Marxist thinkers, Bloch rejects the blueprint version of a perfect future or specific plans to achieve the desired utopia. There is no one right set of steps to the top of the mountain or a heaven on earth. There is no yellow brick road to the emerald city. As one scholar has noted Bloch is a believer in open system

---

[24] Ernst Bloch, *Thomas Münzer als Theologe der Revolution*, 1921.

[25] Wayne Hudson, *The Marxist Philosophy of Ernst Bloch*. (New York: St. Martins Press, 1982):105. *PH* 471–610.

[26] *PH* 794–874; R. Lilienfeld, "Music and Society in the 20th Century: Georg Lukacs, Ernst Bloch, Theodore Adorno," *International Journal of Politics, Culture and Society* 1(1987): 120–146; "The Conscious and Known Activity Within the Not Yet Conscious: The Utopian Function of Art", in *The Utopian Function of Art and Literature* pp. 103–140.also "The Representation of Wish Landscapes in Painting, Opera, and Poetry" pp. 278–293.

Marxism. The Marxist vision is still crucial, but hope has replaced predestination as a key category in achieving this truly great civilization on earth. It is still possible. But not necessary. With this goal human beings can be hopeful of achieving it. Bloch, however, equally emphasizes that this desirable utopia may not be achieved

"Bloch emphasizes that hope is not a guarantee. Hope can only be based on militant optimism which recognizes that the process continues not only the possibility of success but also hazards possibility of destruction".[27]

Before the final section of the *Principle of Hope*, Bloch analyzes incomplete forms of utopias: sociological, medical, technical etc. These goods are not wrong. They are incomplete. The fully just society will include these goods, but it will achieve them in a more just and equal way, both now and in the future.

Bloch discusses seven different partial utopias that envision or try to develop a better more closely perfect human world here on earth. These are ways that human beings have tried envisioned a better world.

1. Social and political thinkers from ancient and medieval times Plato, Joachim of Fiore, Thomas Munzer, Biblical ideas of a land "flowing with milk and honey", natural right thinkers of the enlightenment, etc.[28]
2. Art, Literature and Music.

    Art: da Vinci, Rembrandt, Seurat, Cézanne, Gaugin etc.
    Music and Opera: Beethoven's "Ode to Joy". Mozart's "The Magic Flute", Puccini's La Boehme, or Turandot
    Literature: Romaine de la Rose, Dante's Paradiso, Faust's "Bargen"[29]

3. Philosophical visions: Plato's Republic, Kant's "kingdom of ends", Spinoza's world of complete order.[30]
4. Architectural utopias: ancient temples to the gods, Egyptian tomb architecture, gothic cathedrals, town plans, ideal and real.[31]
5. Geographical utopias: Eden, the isles of the blessed, Atlantis, El Dorado, cities of dreams.[32]

There are two of Bloch's envisioned utopias or parts of a better world that we need to examine more deeply and expand more richly.

First consider the medical utopia.[33] In medicine Bloch envisions that medical knowledge and ability will increase. New forms of treatment for common diseases and medical problems will be developed: medicines, surgery, physical therapy, psychology, and psychiatry, etc. Cures or better treatment for complicated problems

---

[27] *PH* 838–884.
[28] *PH* 699–718.
[29] *PH* 746–798.
[30] *PH* 451–470.
[31] *PH* 455–460.
[32] *PH* 467–470.
[33] *PH* 625–696.

will be found e.g., brain tumors, cancer, spinal fractures, etc. We can hope that medicine will develop better approaches to treating many of the cases we have looked at earlier.

There is a great deal that we have learned about human health and illness in the last century and still much we do not know. The cases we have already presented are examples of this. Medical science has vastly expanded our knowledge of the mentally ill from the time when those with mental problems were thought to be possessed by demons or even from a century ago when Freud thought that being gay was a perversion or that analyzing dreams was a key to treating the mentally ill.

Yet, for all we have learned, much is still a mystery. Schizophrenia, for example, is still largely, a mystery. Successfully treating it even more so. Alzheimer's symptoms are well known but successfully dealing with Alzheimer's or preventing mental decline in the elderly is still very much unknown

Ken Tidwell from Chap. 3 has a well-established diagnosis of schizophrenia. Yet when he refuses necessary surgery, the doctors and the psychologists do not know why or how to persuade him to agree to surgery. When Vicky wants to have her perfectly healthy body deformed Dr. Rogers knows this is wrong but why she desires this is still a mystery. It is also largely unknown how to persuade her not to try to amputate her hand herself.

Margaret Dolan is ill with one of the hardest forms of mental illness to treat, manic depression. The biology of manic depression is not well enough known. Nor is it well-known how to stabilize the highs and the lows. We know much about the brain and are learning more regularly but we do not know enough now to successfully treat Margaret Dolan in a long-term fashion.

All of these medical advances that have happened and those that are still hoped for are grounded in what we know now and what we might know in the future. We already knew about vaccines before we developed a polio vaccine. We knew about the effectiveness of cognitive and behavioral counseling therapies for decades. Originally psychiatrists thought that with the development of psychiatric medications only medication might be needed. Now we know that this one or the other approach was wrong. These approaches are best used together.

Another part of the medical utopia that Bloch presents is to ensure that medical knowledge and care is available to all persons, not just the wealthy or the well-connected. All human beings need medical care. For Bloch, capitalist societies treat people unequally. The best care is for those who have wealth or private insurance. A medical utopia increases medical knowledge and provides both the typical care and the new knowledge universally.[34]

A second utopian project in modernity which Bloch treats extensively and which we need to cover is technology. Before modern times we had dreams and daydreams about Aladdin's lamp, magic potions, various versions of "New Atlantis" or fountains of youth. Now we have actual parts of a technological utopia having been developed or are being developed.

---

[34] *PH* 927–939.

III   71

In the last century telephones and radios have given us access to instant communication over long distances. With satellites we can communicate instantly from the other side of the earth. In World War II Americans had to wait several days to see still pictures of dead or victorious soldiers from faraway in *Life* magazine or we watched newsreels in movie theaters from far away, days after the event.

In Vietnam, footage could be shown on the nightly news. Tragedy was no longer something we read about nor was elation. The whole world watched as Neil Armstrong walked on the moon. "One small step for a man, one giant leap for mankind" As soon as it was announced in Dallas that President Kennedy was declared dead, we saw it announced, as we did when President Nixon announced" I shall resign as president effective at noon tomorrow". Or when President Regan spoke on national television about the disaster of the space shuttle Challenger whose crew members "slipped the steely bands of earth to touch the face of God."

Computer technology and the Internet have only increased our ability to connect to others over long distances. Special events such as the Super Bowl, presidential inaugurations, 9/11 in New York, or other great events such as the installation of a new pope can be seen at the time of the event by anyone around the globe. Some thinkers have thought that we could create robots to do our manual labor.

Automobiles and airplanes have brought our world closer together as persons and in some ways allowed us to see suffering up close. One powerful example of how technology can bring our world closer together is from the mid-1980s. A massive famine developed in the horn of Africa in Somalia and Ethiopia. People were starving by the hundreds of thousands. The rest of the world only read about it. They could not see it in real time. An enterprising reporter from the BBC made his way with great difficulty to the interior, to places where people were starving and dying right before his camera. He shot much footage and brought it out to Bahrain where he uploaded it to BBC headquarters in London. From there it was sent to a major network in New York for broadcast that night.

As the footage was coming in to the newsroom in New York people were stunned and many were in tears. Technology had brought the world together. Technology had also pushed the developed world to mount a massive relief effort that would not have been possible without modern aircraft and other technologies.

Bloch is not the only thinker who has argued that for modernity the ancient quest for the essence of human beings and the nature itself of all reality has been replaced by the Baconian idea of dominating the natural world for human betterment. We are less interested in Aristotle's first and final causes than we are in efficient and material causes, i.e., how an entity works and what it is made of. For example, we are less interested in theoretical mathematics and more interested in how mathematics can enable us to build a more powerful computer. Pure science is most useful and supported by citizens when it can be turned into technology.[35]

The utopias that Bloch treats before the final part of the *Principle of Hope* are grounded in what we know now and what can be known in the future, based on what

---

[35] *PH* 1000–1100.

we know now. They require vigorous study of our world, and more just social systems so that the benefits of technology can be spread more justly: can families have access to the Internet, can those who are poor have access to quality medical care, can cars be designed so that handicapped persons can be easily transported or in some cases drive themselves.

Part five of the *Principle of Hope* is the second longest section of the work. It is about as long as part four. In this section Bloch discusses ways in which human beings have tried to envision final utopias. Bringing together all the partial utopias discussed in part four.

He first treats ancient mythic figures as supposed images of those striving for an end to history or an end of striving e.g., Prometheus, Ulysses, Hercules, etc. He didn't have a long discussion of Goethe's Faust as a literary version of a final universal utopia as is *Don Quixote* who "dreams the impossible dream", but he concludes that these literary visions of Faust and *Don Quixote* were important evidence of humans striving for an ultimate fulfillment. Yet they are incomplete. Just as philosophical visions of human fulfillment in many traditions were ideals in the in the mind, without a temporal earthly foundation.[36]

The two visions of a utopian fulfillment that Bloch treats extensively are music and religion. Music can provide a vision of a completed and fulfilled world. In great operas and symphonies e.g. Beethoven's "ode to joy", Dvorak's New World Symphony, The Magic Flute, The Marriage of Figaro, even Turandot. But while music can enrich and stir the human person to envision a complete *ultimum*, it can only offer a vision of human completeness, not an actual achievement in the real world.[37]

So too is religion. Though Bloch was an atheist, his sympathetic discussion of religion takes almost 200 pages in the English translation. Of course, his ultimate view is that of Feuerbach and the early Marx. God is a projection of humanity. Rather than God creating man, man creates God. Bloch, however, does not disparage religion. He sees in religion a vision of a renewed humanity and a renewed world. It is a vision of human perfection not in the heavens, but in heaven on earth.

He views Christianity as the greatest religion and Christ is the greatest religious founder. For Bloch, Christ is not the son of God but the son of man. Christ's divinity is, in a way, his looking for a just world: his forwardness, his vision of a renewed earth. Christianity takes from Judaism a vision of a land "flowing with milk and honey" and universalizes it. Yahweh was a territorial God and Moses a founder of a specific people. Christ is the beginning of a universal vision of a renewed earth and a new humanity.[38]

Though they give expressions for ourselves and our hope for complete fulfillment, the problem of all these literary, musical, and religious visions of a human fulfillment is that they remain visions not put into practice in the real world. They

---

[36] *PH* 1183–1303.
[37] *PH* 1312 ff.
[38] *PH* 1354 ff.

are expressions of our wishes and dreams and for this they are valuable. But these wishes and dreams need to be put into practice in the real world.

Finally, Bloch believes that a Marxist social, political, intellectual, and artistic order will completely fulfill the human aspirations for fairness, justice, reason, and peace. Whether Bloch is right about this result does not need to be debated here, nor do we need to engage the serious debate about whether Bloch is a faithful follower of Marx. His open system Marxism is obviously not the Marxism of Engels and his followers. The debate about Bloch's Marxism was thoughtful and serious but it need not concern us here.

Bloch's mature work is one of the most powerful recent attempts to organize human life and social, economic, political, and artistic order around the concept of hope. Whether his conclusion is defensible is debatable. But he has shown that hope and aspiration is a core part of human existence. Human beings desire a future that they regard as good. This future is however uncertain. As such, it must be hoped for.

Bloch grounds this hoped for good firmly in this world not either in a divine realm or an eschatological future of a heaven on earth. His hope is firmly in this world. He does not expect any transcendent, divine help to achieve it

When applying Bloch's thinking about hope to medical care we see its power and its limits. Doctors and patients can hope that a particular treatment can care for a particular human person who is sick. They can hope that this medical procedure, surgery or drug treatment can be effective in this situation. Will this surgery remove all the cancer from this person's body? Will this antibiotic rid the infection in this patient's body? if not, the doctor and the patient can hope that a new treatment will be better.

A second sort of medical hope is that new treatments can be developed that will be more effective with less side effects or will be effective in cases where very little effective treatment is available. Can a new treatment for manic depression be developed for difficult cases like that of Margaret Henson? Can a more effective counseling or other therapies be developed to help Vicky not try to cut off her hand?

One important example is the problem of cancer. The first paper in a medical journal describing chemotherapy as a treatment for cancer was published in 1970.[39] Though we have developed many more forms of chemotherapy for many cancers, aside from surgery and radiation, nothing completely new has been developed. Yet doctors and persons with cancer hope that a better way of treating cancer will be found.

All of these medical treatments and new research are based on what we know now and extensions from what we know. They are part of what we can hope for as a better world here on this planet. Religious people may believe that the developments in modern medicine and those that can be expected in the future are the result of divine inspiration. But one does not need to believe that God is involved nor does one need to believe in God to accept the results of modern science. As we have seen in Bloch one can accept religion as an important cultural and historical force, even a positive cultural force, without accepting the central religious belief about the

---

[39] V.T. deVita, E Chu, "History of Cancer Chemotherapy" *Cancer Research*. 68(2008): 8643–8653.

existence of God, God's care for humanity, and/or a transcendent life beyond and after death.

What our analysis in this chapter has shown is a powerful version of temporal hope. A life of justice, peace and human fulfillment that is strictly of this world. This is a modern version of the biblical "land flowing with milk and honey" that God first promised to Abraham and then to the Israelites after they fled from Egyptian slavery.

The Bible presents this as a gift from God. The gift in these cases seems strictly of this world. This gift is not in a transcendent heaven. It is a heaven on earth. What Bloch and other modern versions of this earthly hope desire, without attributing the vision itself or the success hoped for to God. These thinkers want to achieve a richer more stable version of what the fourth century Christians desired.

Chapter 6
Hope and Transcendence

Beyond the temporal hopes for good earthly life and civilization brought about by human effort, exemplified by the work of Ernst Bloch and other non-religious, humanist socialists, and hyper-technologists, there are two versions of religious hope relying on a transcendent power to realize a good beyond human ability to bring it about. The first is the hope of religious groups hoping for a small, transformed part of the world we know, whose transformation is brought about by Divine help: e.g., Hutterites, Moravian Brethren, Diggers, Amish, Quakers, Mennonites, Shakers, early Mormons, etc.[1] This sort of hope for a divinely inspired earthly community will not be a part of our discussion here.

There is another form of religious hope that relies on a transcendent source of power, knowledge and goodness that is not only concerned with small communal life. This chapter examines this transcendent hope as it comes into human caretaking in relation to sickness, suffering, dying, and death. Let us start this analysis with a specific, actual case.

Mr. WK was a 63-year-old divorced white male on dialysis secondary to polycystic renal disease. After being on dialysis for about a year He was admitted to a local hospital with a diagnosis of pericarditis. During this hospitalization he developed a t-6-disc space infection that required removal of the t-6 vertebrae. He consented to all of these procedures. But he then refused stabilization of the spinal column with Harrington Rods. He was transferred from a private hospital to a

---

[1] Tom Scott, *Thomas Munzer: Theology and Revolution in the German Reformation* (London: Macmillan, 1989); Christopher Hill, *The World Turned Upside Down*. (London: Penguin, 1984); Stephen Marini, *Radical Sects of Revolutionary New England*. (Cambridge: Harvard, 1982); George Hunston Williams, *The Radical Reformation*. (Louisville: Westminster John Knox, 1962); Feramorz Fox, *Building the City of God*. (Salt Lake City: Deseret Book, 1974); Leonard Arrington, *Great Basin Kingdom*. (Cambridge: Harvard, 1958).

Veteran's Hospital affiliated with a university medical school after his insurance ran out and the new doctors did not know why he refused the stabilization.

His refusal resulted in paraplegia and a persistent and worsening respiratory infection. Intravenous anti-biotics were only modestly helpful in treating this infection. Pulmonary specialists believed that he had only about 9–10 months left to live. In the ICU his cognitive ability declined rapidly, and psychological evaluations found that he was incapable of making decisions for himself.

When his family, including his elderly mother, divorced father, stepsister, and brother was approached about removing either the respirator or dialysis they would not agree to any removal. They wanted everything done to keep him alive as long as possible. Elsewhere a colleague and I have argued that the doctors in Mr. W. K's case should not just do all that the family members wanted, since that would mean that there would be more suffering for the patient/person.[2]

However, the key family members were deeply religious, evangelical Christians. That is why they called in their minister for comfort and support. So also, was the senior physician overseeing the care of this person. Since the hospital was connected to a medical school, day to day care was provided by residents, also often referred to as "house staff". But their care and the person ultimately responsible for Mr. W.K.'s care was a senior physician who was part of the medical school faculty. This physician was, himself, a deeply religious, evangelical Christian, very similar to the convictions of the family and their pastor.

This physician could work with the pastor. They prayed together for the wellbeing of W.K. They shared their deep faith in a life beyond the bodily grave of W.K. Essentially, for them, W. K's future was in the hands of an all loving, all-powerful, all-knowing God. They could hope that this God would care for W.K. in ways that temporal medicine or loving family and friends could not. That good would triumph over sadness, sickness, and despair.

I   Gabriel Marcel: Hope and Transcendence

In the twentieth century no philosopher/theologian has written more deeply about hope and transcendence than the French thinker Gabriel Marcel. It is to his work we now turn for a richer understanding of hope and transcendence in the face of sickness, suffering, uncertainty and death, conditions that Marcel himself might refer to as "evil". Marcel's work is so multifaced, including articles, books, and plays that

---

[2] I have analyzed the moral issues in this case elsewhere. Richard Sherlock and C. Mary Dingus, "Families and the Gravely Ill: Roles, Rules, and Rights", *Journal of the American Geriatric Society*. 33(1985): 121–124.

we can only treat and employ some of it here. We shall employ his work that focuses on hope and God, especially in the cases just noted as "evil".[3]

II Problem and Mystery

One of Marcel's central distinctions is crucial in understanding hope and transcendence in the face of human suffering. This is the distinction between a problem and a mystery. Human beings live in a broken world of sickness, tragedy, uncertainty, and death. One of the central ways we engage this broken world is to view it as a series of problems.[4]

Problems are a way of seeing the world as a discrete series of events or engagements with other persons, events, groups, and nature that I can manage or "solve". As this is being written it is snowing outside. Thus, getting home is a problem that I must solve. If I am to get home safely specific things will have to be done. I will have to brush the snow off my car in the parking lot. I will have to drive home more slowly. I may find it preferable to take another route where there will be fewer cars on the road. By taking these steps I can "solve" the problem of getting home safely with it snowing.

In another personal example, I have diabetes which was diagnosed for me about 15 years ago. This is a problem that can be managed. I cannot eat things that are sweet or sugary. Fortunately, I have always liked coffee black. But I have had to give up ice cream, cake, and cookies. I must test my blood sugar daily and inject insulin twice a day. I must see my doctor regularly for lab work examining my kidney function and long-term blood glucose level. My diabetes is a problem for me, my doctor,

---

[3] Marcel's works:

Being and Having trans. Katharine Farrer (Westminster, UK.: Dacres Press, 1949) BH

The Mystery of Being vol 1 Reflections and Mystery trans. G.S. Fraser (London: The Harvill Press, 1951) MB 1

The Mystery of Being Vol 2 Faith and Reality trans. Rene Hauge (London: The Havrill Press, 1951) MB 2

Homo Viator: Introduction to the Metaphysics of Hope. trans. Emma Crawford (New York: Harper Torchbooks, 1962) HV

Man Against Mass Society. trans G.S. Fraser (Chicago: Henry Regnery, 1962). MAM

Philosophy of Existentialism trans. Manya Harari (London: Harvill Press, 1948) PE.

[4] For this distinction see BH 100–126; MV 68–69; also see Kenneth Gallagher, *The Philosophy of Gabriel Marcel* (New York: Fordham University Press, 1962): 30–49; Thersa Tobin "Toward an Apology of Mysticism: Knowing God as a Mystery", *International Philosophical Quarterly.* 50(2010): 221–241; Simone Ploudre "Gabriel Marcel and the Mystery of Suffering" *Anuavia Filosophia* 38(2005): 575–596; *K.R.Hanley,* ed. *Gabriel's Perspectives on the Broken World.* (Milwaukee: Marquette University Press, 1998); Gene Reeves, "The Idea of Mystery in the Philosophy of Gabriel Marcel" in Paul Schilpp and Lewis Hahn eds. The Philosophy of Gabriel Marcel. (La Salle, Ill.: Open Court,1984): 245–272.

and my family. This problem in my broken world can be solved by me, with help from my doctor, family, and friends.[5]

Human life is dominated or consumed by problems. When my car breaks down, how do I get to work in the morning? How do I get my kids to stop playing video games and go outside and exercise? How do I explain a complicated problem in medieval philosophy to undergraduates e.g., what is the relation between philosophy and faith in Avicenna? How do I revise a paper so it can be published? How do I help my wife get well after an illness or help her find a better job?

Much medicine, especially modern medicine, is generally understood as a series of discrete problems. With the enormous growth of medical specialties in the last century medical practice has become a series of specialists who "solve" a series of discrete "problems": e.g., migraines, twisted knees, kidney failure, hearing loss, intestinal blockage, breast cancer. These and thousands of other "problems" are "solved" by specialists, e.g., neurologists, oncologists, audiologists, orthopedic surgeons, etc.[6]

Of course, in these cases hope is still central. Will the orthopedic surgeon be able to repair the knee so that the patient can walk without pain or a walker? With modern x-rays and CAT scans the doctor can give the patient a much better prognosis but hope still is important. A nephrologist has several treatments he or she can use to treat someone with damaged kidneys. But the nephrologist must hope that they can be effective in any particular patient. With improvements in chemotherapy the oncologist can successfully treat childhood cancer better than ever before. But the uncertainty remains. The patient, the patient's family, and the doctor must hope that the "problem" of childhood leukemia can be successfully solved in the case of this specific child.

In the cases we have seen in Chaps. 2 and 3 there are problems to be solved. In Chap. 2 Mark Davis' doctor and family must hope that he can be persuaded to have surgery. The surgery is routine for an experienced physician. The problem is to overcome Mark's resistance, which is based on patently false beliefs. In Vicki's case the problem is her abnormal desire to damage her normal, healthy body. In these cases, there is no uncertainty about what the result should be. There may be underlying causes that lead to the problems for the persons and physicians in each of these cases, but the doctors, patients, and families have a discrete problem to solve.

So also, are the cases in Chap. 3. Chuck's prostate cancer is a problem to be solved with surgery and perhaps chemotherapy. A more difficult problem is to also solve the other problems, in his case, preserving urinary continence and the possibility of marital intimacy for Chuck and Joan. Though these goals are more difficult to achieve, achieving them is a specific problem to be solved. Chuck, Joan, and

---

[5] M. Regina Castro m.d. *Mayo Clinic: The Diabetes Book* 3rd ed. (Rochester MN: Mayo Clinic).

[6] cf. Paul Starr, *The Social Transformation of Medicine.* (New York: Basic Books, 1982); Stanley Reiser, *Medicine, and the Reign of Technology.* (Cambridge: Cambridge University press, 1978); George Weisz, "The Emergence of Medical Specialization in the 19th Century" *Bulletin of the History of Medicine.* 77(2003):536–577.

II Problem and Mystery

Dr. Frazier must hope that these problems can be solved. But they remain problems. If they are solved, all three persons will know.

The three goals of treatment for Dan Kelly are also specific and discrete. They are problems with a solution. Dan, his wife, and Dr. Flandro will know whether these problems have been solved. They must hope that these problems can be successfully solved. But there is no mystery in what the solution to these problems will be.

Of course, in medicine each patient is unique, even physically. However, physically the uniqueness of each patient is relatively minor. This is why, physically, medicine can be regarded as a science. As a science, we can perform the same operation on different patients the same way all the time. We can prescribe the same medicine for Joe's high blood pressure and Jane's. Millions of other persons can inject the same insulin I inject every day, because they have the same physical needs I do.

Marcel himself writes of this fact about problems in general in a passage that seems specific for this point in medicine.

"When I am dealing with a problem, I am trying to discover a solution that becomes common property, that can, at least in theory, be rediscovered by anybody at all. But…this idea of a validity for "anybody at all" or of a thinking in general has less and less application the more deeply one penetrates the inner courts of philosophy"[7] In philosophy, formal logic works out the same for anybody at any time and place. Affirming the consequent is always wrong.

This fact of broad application is seen in the way the FDA requires studies showing that a new drug is effective for either the general public, e.g., a new pain relief pill or for a part of the population e.g., an antidepressant or a new drug for an irregular heartbeat. The FDA does not require that the drug is effective for every person with a specific medical problem. But it must be effective for many or most. It cannot be effective for just one person. It must also be safe for most of those for whom it is prescribed.[8]

As experienced clinicians know and as argued for powerfully by Richard Clarke Cabot, however, caring for a sick person is more than solving a series of discrete problems. One person's heart problem will be the same as another's, with the same physical manifestation. But as Cabot so eloquently argued a person as a patient is more than a series of problems that can be solved with a new drug or a new procedure that can be used to treat many others. Each suffering soul that requires both a doctor and a pastor, priest or rabbi is different and healing their suffering soul requires reaching their suffering whole person in a manner different than anyone else. Furthermore, each person's social situation is unique to that person. Their family life, their employment, their physical living space is different. So too is their

---

[7] MB 1: 213.

[8] *Center for Drug Evaluation and Development and Approval Process*. Available at FDA.Gov

education, the social groups they belong to, and especially their religious faith. Patients are first persons.[9]

To treat and care for the whole person is much more and fundamentally different than solving a series of problems because the human person is more than a series of things. And life is more than a series of events.

Caring for the whole person in this way brings us to Marcel's concept of a "mystery" which is fundamentally different than a problem. A problem is an object that can be analyzed and solved like an auto mechanic who must fix a specific problem in a specific car or an airline pilot who must fly a specific airplane on a specific route.

Caring for another is different because a person is not an object like an airplane or an automobile. Doctors and nurses do perform mechanical tasks with patients: checking blood pressure, blood glucose level, blood oxygen or a surgery to remove an intestinal blockage etc. In these cases, blood pressure or eyesight is an object that can be analyzed, and problems solved.

But caring for the whole person is deeper than problem solving. Caring for a person engages the caretaker and the cared for in a comprehensive relationship where two persons have a mysterious bond of care, compassion, and love. Also, there is physical support and obligations. When my mentally ill wife buys something online that we do not really need, I have an obligation to pay for it. When she cannot drive, I must drive us to church, to her doctor's appointment, and to the store. We have been married for decades. We care for each other. We are committed to each other "for better or worse, for richer or poorer, in sickness and in health". In a real sense, her sickness is my sickness, her happiness is my happiness. When she grieves, I grieve.

Our relation is what Marcel would call a mystery. It cannot be reduced to a checklist. In caretaking a mystery transforms both the caregiver and the one cared for. The caretaker learns more about themselves than they knew before, and more than a third party could see or grasp from outside the relationship as an object. The person cared for realizes the goodness of the caretaker and his or her deep gratitude for a world in which there are those who are caregivers, persons who engage others with faith in a reality where good ultimately triumphs; hope that this good will be realized for this relationship. And love of the persons for each other and for the power that can light the darkness of what Marcel calls a "broken world" so we can see the good.[10]

A mystery is "engaged" it is not "solved". A mystery engages the whole person not just a part. It transforms both persons as whole persons. These persons have physical bodies and physical attributes e.g., hair color, height, right or left handedness. They have beliefs and commitments, some are trivial, some are basic or foundational such as religious beliefs for many people. To use an analogy, they are plants

---

[9] cf. Richard Clarke Cabot *What Men Live By: Work, Play, Love, Worship*. (New York: Houghton Mifflin 1914).
[10] PE 10–20; Gabriel Marcel, "The Mystery of the Family" in HV: 62–90.

II Problem and Mystery 81

that have grown up in one garden and now in this new relationship they must grow in a different garden.

Because they are human persons not just plants, they are open to something different than they have been before. As persons they are able to grow in new and different gardens with new and different people, as converts from one religion to another do or families moving from one country to another with a different culture and a different language. They change while remaining the same. This stability and change is more than solving a problem. It is a development that is a mystery.[11]

A good example of this is from the life of a late friend of mine. The family came to America from Hungary in the 1920s. The parents hoped for a better life for them and their children than they could expect in war ravaged Europe. His father took a job in the emerging auto industry in Detroit and the family prospered in the new country.

The family was deeply Catholic, so they attended mass every week at a parish with priests from Hungary, where the congregants were Hungarian. In the summer the priests had the children come in the morning 3 days a week to the church. Here they kept their culture and language alive. They learned Hungarian history, sang Hungarian songs, read Hungarian children's books. At noon the mothers would prepare a Hungarian meal.[12]

This developed the children as whole persons whose personhood is not found in manuals or reduced to a checklist. Their relationship with each other, the priests and their parents was not like someone wiring a new house or fixing a leaky faucet. The relation of the children with each other, with the adults and with the priests, transformed both. In Marcel's word this transformational relationship is a mystery.

Another example of this same transformative mystery of persons in relation involves medicine directly and a former student at my university. This young man wanted to go to medical school from an early age, which he was able to do. Before graduating from my university, he had spent 2 years in Costa Rica as a missionary for the LDS Church and was fluent in Spanish. Unlike many medical students he wanted to be a family practice physician. He wound up practicing in Texas in a large city on the border with Mexico. In this city there were several large employers producing a variety of consumer goods. For most of the employees their native language was Spanish.

These employers joined together and funded a primary care clinic with four family practice doctors, a small laboratory, and an x-ray machine. If employees or their family members needed care, they could go to this clinic and pay a modest co-pay. If they sought care elsewhere, except in an emergency, they paid the full cost. These doctors could refer patients to specialists as needed.

Some of the doctors in this clinic knew basic Spanish. But the former student from my university was in high demand because of his fluency in Spanish,

---

[11] J.B O'Malley, *The Fellowship of Being: An Essay on the Concept of the Person in the Philosophy of Gabriel Marcel*. (The Hague: Martinus Nijhoff, 1966).

[12] Hungarian food contains much meat, much cabbage, and the spice paprika is used generously.

especially with mothers and their children. They would come in and he would speak to them in the colloquial Spanish they were used to and address the children by their first name. He came to know them as persons, not just patients. He could talk to them about their lives, not just their illness, e.g., "how do you like school?", "what is your favorite food?". If they were older, he would ask "Do you have a girlfriend or boyfriend?"

To him they were persons, not problems. As persons his relationship with them was more than a problem to be solved like a sore throat or a broken leg. In Marcel's sense they came together as persons in a mystery, knowing the relationship was good but not knowing what sort of good would appear at each visit. When some of his long-time patients/persons knew that it was his tenth anniversary at the clinic they had a party for him and his family at the end of the day.

III Faith

How in deeply understanding a mystery we are led to think about faith and hope and the transcendent ground of both.

In my view, developed from Marcel, faith, what Marcel refers to as fidelity, is a threefold concept.[13] In the beginning it can be understood as a sort of "keeping one's word", a commitment to follow through with what a person told others they were going to do, e.g., meet someone for lunch, call someone at a certain time, attend a meeting. I may not want to attend or do not think I need to attend this meeting. But the other committee members have faith that I will attend, and I have faith that they will also attend. A client has faith that a lawyer can get him a large settlement from a company whose product the client believes has injured him or her. Another client believes that their lawyer can enable them to be found innocent when charged with a crime. Patients have faith that their doctor can solve their specific medical problem. The patient does not know. He or she has faith that this problem can be solved by this person.

In each of the instances we just noted the professionals also have faith. The doctor has faith in his ability to heal. The lawyers have faith in their abilities to defend a person accused of a crime or obtain a large settlement. The head of the committee has faith that the members will attend the meeting so that what the committee needs to accomplish can be done.

To return to *Equus*, Martin Dysart has strong faith in his ability to successfully heal Alan Strang i.e., to solve his problem. "I'll heal the rash on his body. I'll erase the welts cut into his mind by flying manes. When that's done, I'll send him on a nice mini-scooter off into the normal world where animals are treated properly…you wont gallop anymore Alan. Horses will be quite safe. You'll save your pennies every

---

[13] BH 41; also, the essay in HV "Obedience and Fidelity" pp. 118–127.

week till you can change that scooter for a car and put the odd fifty pence on the nags."[14]

In the *Plague*, Rieux and Castel have faith in their diagnosis that the cause of the sickness, suffering and death in Oran is the actual plague. They also have faith in their ability to care for those persons who are suffering and dying every day.[15]

This sort of temporal faith is in a way twofold. First, it can be faith in one event or action. I can have faith that other members of the committee will come to this meeting. Furthermore, I can have faith that the committee will accomplish what needs to be done, e.g. hire a new faculty member or appoint a new department head. When a major league baseball manager calls in a relief pitcher from the bullpen, he has faith that this pitcher, in this situation, will perform as required. I can have faith that in a local election good candidates will be elected to the city council.

These and millions of other cases are faith in a specific event. In a second way this sort of faith need not be limited to a specific time and place. The baseball manager must have faith in this pitcher's ability for more than one situation. A basketball coach must have faith in his team for more than one game, If the manager or the coach did not have this faith, they would replace their players with players in whom he could have faith.

As a member of the committee, I must have faith that the work of this committee over a long period of time is worth my time and effort. When I am driving, I must have faith that other drivers will obey the traffic rules not just in one moment, but in every moment. I must also have faith that not just some drivers will stop at red lights and stay in their lanes but that every driver will stop at every red light. In none of these cases do the persons involved know that the result they desire will come about. Neither the manager nor the coach knows whether their team can win a particular game or have certain hitter strike out. There are enough times when the pitcher doesn't get the hitter out, the team doesn't play well, or the driver doesn't stop that faith is required in these sorts of cases. Finally, I have been on enough dysfunctional committees that I must have faith that this committee will do what it is supposed to do.

The third part of the general concept of faith is exemplified in the case we started this chapter with. The pastor of W. K's family and the senior physician who was ultimately responsible for his care share a deep faith in a transcendent power who can and has intervened, in situations just like this. They cannot know that this power, i.e., God, exists as I know that I have a pen in my hand or that today there is rain outside where I am. Nor can the senior physician know the existence of the Christian God, as surely as he knows what is wrong with W.K. He must have faith in a personal God and this God's ability to intervene in cases just like this.[17]

The pastor, the family, and the physician also have faith that there is a sort of existence for individuals beyond the bodily grave of Mr. W.K. and any of us. Since they cannot journey to this "place" before death and a bring us a first-hand report,

---

[14] Equus: 124.
[15] Plague: 47–51.

neither they nor we can know about this existence the way we can know about the surface of the moon from Neil Armstrong, or Englishmen could know about the Sandwich Islands from Capitan James Cook.[16] The family, the pastor, and the physician must have a faith in the existence of such a "place" and in God.

Martin Dysart wants this sort of faith in a transcendent source of meaning and spiritual engagement. He knows he lacks such a faith. His lack torments him. Alan Strang has a faith in and experience of the sort of God that Martin desires and lacks. Martin is troubled that if he cures Alan from the twisted faith he has, he will destroy Alan's ability to have true, strong faith. Alan may go to a worship service and not actually worship anything at all.

Chuck Gardner and his wife Joan have a deep faith in the biblical God, who, as we have noted, saved human life on earth with Noah and his family, parted the Red Sea, kept the jar of flour full for the woman who fed Elijah, brought Lazarus back from the dead, and resurrected Jesus. Whether these events happened is not an issue here. Chuck and Joan have faith that they did, and in a God that brought them about.

Claire Darlington, in her condition, cannot express her faith. But her family can. They have faith in a God who can intervene at any place and time. These are not just the biblical miracles we just noted. These are contemporary miracles, the claims of which are scrutinized by medical experts to see if there is any explanation other than divine intervention for the result, e.g., healing a sick person or saving the life of a person who is dying.[17]

Claire's family and, so far as we know, Claire herself have faith in such a God who has the knowledge and ability to intervene in the material world He created, an intervention that has happened and is happening now. Claire's family and the priests do not know why or how God intervenes. But they have faith in such a God.

The infectious disease specialist at the university hospital, Dr. Karen Steel, also has faith in a God, much like the God in which Chuck and Joan have faith. Thus, she can have faith of three results: (1) that God will intervene and save Claire's life, (2) that a better life awaits Claire after the earthly grave, and (3) that she, Dr. Steel, will learn something that will help other sick persons. The family, the priests and Dr. Steel have faith that good will triumph in this imperfect "broken world".

Whether Linda Janko, the Jehovah's Witness, has faith in such a god we do not know. It seems clear that her sister does. Her sister vocally professes a belief in such a God who requires real personal sacrifice and will reward it in the afterlife. The emergency room doctor has faith in a God who has required such a commitment from saints, martyrs, and ordinary persons in his own Catholic faith.

---

[16] The sandwich islands, now known as Hawaii, were discovered by British explorer James Cook in 1778.

[17] In the Catholic church to be recognized as a miracle in the process of becoming recognized as a saint the event must be examined by a panel of experts assembled by the Vatican. They must judge that there is no know way that this event could have happened without Divine intervention. For examining the general question of miracles see Graham Twelftree ed. *The Cambridge Companion to Miracles*. (London: Cambridge University Press, 2009).

In each of these cases faith is a faith in a transcendent power that can and has intervened in the course of nature or can require suffering from which true good will flow. For those with such faith the ultimate source of a person's faith is unknown fully. Persons are often raised in families and communities that ground them in such a faith but why they keep such a faith as they grow is only partially understood.

But the faith we have seen in these cases, as examples of what Marcel calls "fidelity", is more objective and less personal than what becomes hope. For Claire's family their faith in a God who can and has intervened is partially grounded in the study of experts who examine medical data with a skeptical, objective attitude. Only after all natural explanations have been eliminated do they conclude that God might have intervened. In Marcel's words they study it as a problem to be solved, not a mystery to be lived and accepted.

In these cases, the person can say:

I have faith that X exists
X is God
X can intervene in the course of nature
Therefore, X can intervene here

Though God is different than any other person or entity, what makes this structurally different than:

I desire car X
I have faith that I can afford X
Therefore, I will buy X
Or following Augustine
I have faith that X exists
Satin is X
Satin can lead people to do evil
Therefore, for me, Satin exists and can lead me to do evil.

Faith of the type held by Chuck and Joan, Dr. Steele, Claire's family, priests, and Mr. WK's, family, pastor, and the senior physician, goes beyond merely being impersonal. It is a faith in a personal God who can intervene in nature to alter events and bring about a result that empirical science, medical judgment, or previous study could not have predicted.

IV Hope

Hope in the types of cases that we have before us is different. In cases like these hope builds on faith. But it goes beyond faith. Like faith, hope also has both temporal, ordinary uses and uses where it points beyond the temporal to the transcendent.

Marcel notes that in many cases hope points to something very ordinary. "I hope that my friend can have lunch with me tomorrow". "I hope that my son did well on his CPA exam yesterday". "I hope that my daughter did well on the MCAT exam on Saturday". Like faith, these temporal hopes can and often are hopes for some specific temporal good. "I hope that Mary does well in this specific, difficult math class". "I hope that Sharon gets into Princeton". "I hope that my favorite candidate gets elected to be the next mayor". "I hope that students in my medieval philosophy class will understand Maimonides' negative theology."[18]

To return to our committee meeting example. I can have faith that all the other members will attend. I can have faith that the committee will achieve what it is supposed to achieve in this meeting.

To say "I hope" is different. "I hope that others will attend" is a statement of uncertainty. I do not know or have faith, but I desire their attendance. I do not know that the committee will accomplish what it is supposed to accomplish, but I desire this result. As such I hope that it will.

Like faith, there is a second sort of temporal hope for a result longer and broader than one event. I can hope that this committee will function to examine more cases of academic fraud or dishonesty. I can hope that after a terrible war there will be more than a moment of peace, but that there will be an era of peace. When my wife is seriously ill, I can hope that she will recover and remain well for a long period of time.

This second form of hope is not fundamentally different from the first. It is only an extension of the first. I hope my wife is healthy today and for all or at least many days to come. I hope that teaching Maimonides in my medieval philosophy class was understood by my students in this class and the next time I teach it and the next after that. The manager hopes that this pitcher is successful in this game, at this point and in many other games at other points.

These hopes of both the first immediate kind and the longer term temporal kind for a result continuing in the future are what Marcel calls "I hope of a very low order". In these cases, such as Marcel's example of hoping to have lunch with a friend, I desire a result, but it is not certain that this result will happen.[19]

Though they may appear similar, hope, for Marcel, is different than optimism. The optimist generally expects that what he or she desires will come about; "everything will turn out for the best—you'll see". Two elements distinguish this from hope, especially hope in cases of suffering, sickness, and despair. The optimists seem to know what for them is really good, i.e. desirable. Of this the optimist has no doubt.

Secondly, while they cannot know for certain, like they can know that the temperature where they are is 70°, they expect that what they desire will come to pass. Optimists expect a specific result that they desire and believe is good. To quote Marcel "The optimist is he who has a firm conviction or in certain cases just a vague feeling that things tend to turn out for the best."[20]

---

[18] HV:22; BH 91ff.
[19] HV 22–23.
[20] HV 27–28.

IV Hope   87

But hope, especially of the sort we are about to consider is a hope whose nature is mysterious and whose success is also mysterious.

These examples I have given are cases of this sort of hope that Marcel would refer to as "hope that X". In a powerful passage Marcel writes of a very different sort of hope.

"Now let us suppose, on the contrary, that I am going through a time of trial, either in my private affairs or in that of the group to which I belong. I long for the deliverance which would bring the trial to an end. The "I hope" in all its strength is directed towards salvation. It really is a matter of my coming out of a darkness in which I am at present plunged and which may be the darkness of illness, separation, exile, or slavery. It is obviously impossible in such cases to separate the 'I hope' from a certain type of situation of which it is really a part. Hope is situated within the framework of the trial, not only corresponding to it but constituting our being's veritable response."[21]

This darkness can be despair at one's own situation, one's disability or disease. For Marcel the human person does not seek or desire to live in darkness. In these cases of illness or disability, being a permanent invalid or handicapped in some other way the soul "wants to see the shining of that veiled mysterious light which we feel sure, without any analysis, illumines the very center of hope's dwelling place."[22]

For Marcel, in the cases of sickness and suffering which is our focus here, hope is a mystery not a problem. The person, the family, the medical experts, and the pastors or priests hope for a good which is, in Marcel's view, a light shining in the broken world, that lights a way forward in the darkness.

This light is not like turning on a light switch or lighting a lantern. These acts are a solution to the problem of a dark room. The darkness of sickness and suffering is different. Thus, in these cases, the hope here is a mystery that defies problem solving. Of course, in these cases there are problems to be solved. A person who cannot feed themselves must be fed. An invalid must be bathed and helped to the bathroom. But a person is more than a series of bodily functions. A person is a whole that is more complex and larger than a sum of parts. As such, hope, for the person, is a hope that good will triumph over the evil of a broken world. How this good will be realized or what this good will be is a mystery.

As we have already seen, to say that "I hope" means that I am not certain but that I desire a certain result because I believe that this result is good. Faith is a belief that something exists or will come to pass in the future, whether this result is good or bad.

For Marcel, and this writer, I begin by hoping that some specific result that I desire and believe is good will come about. I do not know how or when. Ultimately, however, I hope that good will triumph over evil in this broken world.

This triumph is a mystery. The person who hopes does not know and cannot know how or when. But as Marcel says this foundational hope is "I hope in Thee for

---

[21] HV p 24.
[22] HV 26.

us." Hope in this sense remains a mystery. Its ground the "Thee", what he also calls as an "Absolute Thou", is only partially known. How and why this "Thee" enables good to come about is a mystery that goes beyond reason, a mystery that we can experience but never fully understand. As Marcel himself says "hope is a mystery not a problem."[23]

To see the difference between faith and hope consider driving a car. My driving a car on a street requires that I have faith that other drivers know the rules of the road and will follow them. This is a general principle in which drivers have faith. The experience of most drivers provides reasonable grounds for this faith. In a specific instance I must hope that a specific driver will follow the rules in a specific situation, e.g., when the road is slippery this driver will go more slowly or will allow more time to break at a stop sign. I can have faith in the driver's general knowledge and ability and hope that the driver's knowledge and ability are used here.

Ultimately, for Marcel and for many of those in the cases we have seen this fundamental hope points to a transcendence of a world of solvable problems and leads to a good that cannot be calculated and to a source of this good that must be experienced not argued for. In these cases, and many others, the persons involved must have faith that such a source exists and hope that it will triumph over the broken world in this case.

For Marcel hope is grounded in and grounds a conviction that the future is open not closed. The deepest hope for the triumph of the good requires us to let go of what we may have so that we can see the future as open, for something more experientially beautiful and truly good. Holding on to what we have limits the freedom of an open future. As he writes: "being and having in our society teaches us how to take possession of things, when it should rather initiate us in the art of letting go. For there is neither freedom nor real life without an apprenticeship in letting go." Hope is grounded in a conviction that beyond all tabulations and inventories a "mysterious principle" is working for me. The freest person he notes is the one "with the most hope."[24]

In the cases we have seen in Chaps. 2 and 3 some of the patients, families and physicians are religious in the typical or usual sense. For Chuck and Joan, Claire and her family and Dr. Steel, as well as the family and physician we started this chapter with, their faith leads them to believe that, in Marcel's words that the "future in open". God has the power to bring about a good that they cannot know but can only hope for.

In all the cases we have seen, the doctors have faith in the correctness of the diagnosis, in their plan for treatment, and in their ability to successfully follow the plan they have laid out.

---

[23] HV 54–56.
[24] BH; HV 46–48: also L.A. Bain, "Marcel's Logic of Freedom in Proving the Existence of God," *International Philosophical Quarterly*. 9(1969): 177–204; Joe McCown, *Availability: Gabriel Marcel and the Phenomenology of Human Openness*. (Missoula, Montana: Scholars Press, 1978).

But all these doctors must hope that for them and for the persons who are their patients, the world is open, no matter how despairing and closed it may appear.

Even in the most desperate situations doctors must hope that the world is open, not closed. If it were closed it would be irrational and useless to go forward. In Claire Darlington's case Dr. Steel expected her to die that night. Dr. Gupta expects her to die in surgery. These were prognoses that they regarded as highly likely. However, this was not a fact like the sunrise tomorrow at a specific time or even Claire's blood pressure when it was taken. Claire's earthly future was open. If it were closed, they would not have tried to save her life. Even though Dr. Gupta is not religious in the traditional sense he must view the world as open. If it is open, then his hope that for Claire good can triumph over despair is not irrational. He must hope that Claire's life can be saved. Thus, in Percival's words, he is a "minister of hope" for Claire, her son, and her family.

Of course, Claire, her family, and Dr. Steel have another form of hope in an open world. This hope is that Claire's future is open even beyond the earthly grave. This is a hope in a transcendent realm where complete fulfillment and happiness are permanent. This is the place where good permanently triumphs over despair in this broken world.

Even Dr. Gupta, who does not believe in this transcendent world, must hope for something beyond saving Claire's life. He must hope that in operating on Claire his surgical skill in very difficult cases will improve, i.e., for his profession, the future is open. Secondly, he and Dr. Steel must hope that when the signs and symptoms that Claire has exhibited appear in another person, they and the doctors in her hometown will have a better idea of what the medical problems of this new patient/person are and can intervene earlier. Thus, even Dr. Gupta is a "minister of hope" to himself and his profession.

In Linda Janko's case Dr. Masely can only act with hope, no matter which way he acts. If does not save Linda's life he must hope that for her the future is open in another existence, similar to the paradise where he believes that saints who were martyrs in his own Catholic faith exist. In this way he must hope that a transcendent existence will triumph over this broken world. If he operates and saves Linda's life, he must hope that her family, friends, and religious community can welcome her, even if some of them disapprove of what he did. Dr. Masely must hope that for her the future is open both for her physical life and for her spiritual life.

In the cases we just looked at and those of Chuck and Joan, and W.K. some of the doctors and patients are religious in the typical sense. Some are not. In the case of Margaret Dolan, neither Margaret, her husband Don nor Dr. Henkson are religious in the manner of Chuck and Joan or W. K's family and the senior physician responsible for his care.

Yet Dr. Henkson must ground his continuing care for Margaret in a hope that good will triumph over her and Don's suffering and often despair in this imperfect and "broken" world. Treating successfully her manic depression is an elusive goal. Success will be measured in small steps. Yet Dr. Henkson cannot care for Margaret and her relationship with Don unless he hopes for a result that he cannot know or predict. For Dr. Henkson, Margaret's future must be open, no matter how closed it may appear for Margaret, Don, and, at times, Dr. Henkson.

V Belif, Faith and Hope

Faith essentially connects to belief. Some of the persons in our cases have strong beliefs about "miraculous" events in the Bible, e.g., saving the world with Noah, parting the Red Sea or raising Lazarus from the dead. To say that these patients, pastors, physicians, and families had faith that these events happened is not fundamentally different than saying that they believed that these events happened.

For many of these sorts of beliefs persons can give reasons for their beliefs. For the existence of Troy and the trojan war the person who believes can rely on substantial evidence from archeologists that Troy actually existed and was destroyed by a massive invasion.[25] In the case of the flood the believer can rely on substantial archeological evidence of a massive flood in the near east at the end of the last ice age. This flood would have covered all the "world" that the writer of *Genesis* and the *Epic of Gilgamesh* knew.[26] In other cases we have good grounds to believe that something did happen that we wish did not, e.g., cannibalism among the Anasazi in the southwest.[27]

To say that one believes that Troy existed, that Moses was a real person, or that there was a flood is not structurally different than having faith that these persons and events actually existed or happened.

The same point is true about faith in God. There is no fundamental difference between:

I have faith that God exists.
And
I believe that God exists.

When the theist is asked why he has faith in the existence of God. He or she can give reasons. The theist might offer the ontological argument from Anselm and as it was made more powerful by Leibniz, Hartshorne, Plantinga and others.[28]

---

[25] Susan Allen, *Finding the Walls of Troy*. (Berkley: University of California Press, 1999); Jane Carter and Susan Morris eds. *The Ages of Homer*. (Austin: University of Texas Press, 1995).

[26] William Ryan and Walter Pitman *Noah's Flood*. (New York: Simon and Schuster, 2000).

[27] Brian Billman, Patricia Lambert, Banks Leonard, "Cannibalism, Warfare, and Drought in the Mesa Verde Region During the Twelfth Century A.D", *American Antiquity*. 65(2000): 145–178: Patricia Lambert, Brian Billman, Banks Leonard, "Explaining Variability in Mutilated Bone Assemblages in the American Southwest: A Case Study from the Southern Piedmont of Sleeping Ute Mountain Colorado" *International Journal of Osteoarcheology*. 10(2000): 49–64.

[28] M. Charlesworth, *Anselm's Proslogion*. (London: Oxford University Press, 1965); Charles Hartshorne, *Anselm's Discovery*. (La Salle Ill.: Open Court, 1965); Alvin Plantinga, *The Nature of Necessity*. (London: Oxford University Press, 1974).

V   Belif, Faith and Hope

The theist might offer Aquinas' "five ways" or parts of them that have been strengthened by modern science: the "first cause" argument that has been made stronger by the development of "big bang" cosmology or the design argument that has been enriched by modern genetics and by "fine tuning" argument in the "big bang" cosmology.[29]

Whether these arguments are sound is highly contested. But the theist has arguments to justify his faith that God exists.

Even more ordinary uses of the term "faith" are not fundamentally different than belief.

To say, "I have faith that if we hire this person for this job, it will be done well" is no different than saying "I believe that if we hire this person the job will get done well." Or "I have faith that this car is the best one for me to buy" is no different than saying "I believe that this car is the best one for me to buy". In each case the person can give reasons for their judgment.

Hope is different. As we have seen hope rests on desire and uncertainty. As Augustine noted I can believe or have faith that Satan exists. But to say that "I hope that Satan exists" is a misuse of language. Given the brokenness of the world, the evidence of evil in the world is a reasonable ground for believing or having faith that Satan exists.

A person may have faith that God exists. But a person must hope for God's help in a specific case. Having faith in a God who can intervene is different than saying "I hope he will intervene here."

The role of hope in medicine is fundamental. As we have seen in the cases presented here hope must ground what doctors do or don't do. In the final analysis doctors, patients/persons, family, and friends must hope that good can triumph over evil in this "broken world". How or when good will triumph is what Marcel calls a mystery, as is the source of this triumph. To hope for this triumph is to see the future as open, not closed.

Much of modern medicine can be viewed as problem solving. The person being cared for, however, is more than collection of problems. All medical professionals must seek the good of the person for whom they care. Sometimes this good is obvious, e.g., removing an intestinal blockage or putting in a pacemaker. At other times this good is either not so obvious or it is uncertain whether this good can be achieved. As such, hope that good can triumph in the "broken world" that medical professionals wrestle with daily is essential to the practice of medicine. This is a hope that goes beyond science and rational arguments like those for the existence of God. This is a hope that is grounded in the openness of the world that empirical study cannot fully understand.

Over two centuries ago Thomas Percival's claim that doctors are a "minister of hope" was profoundly right, more so than he realized even in a much more

---

[29] CF. Stephen Barr, *Modern Science and Ancient Faith*. (Notre Dame: Notre Dame University Press, 2004); William Dembski and Michael Ruse eds. *Debating Design*. (London: Cambridge University Press, 2004); Frank Salisbury, *The Case for Divine Design*. (Springville, UT.: Cedar Fort, 2006).

scientifically advanced era of medical practice. His practical advice about how to sustain this hope was seriously wrong. But doctors who do not hope for themselves, their patients, and their practice do not care for person they care for now and those they will care for in the future.

Cases

Charles Gardner
Clair Darlington
Dan Kelly
Ken Tidwell
Linda Janko
Margaret Dolan
Mark Wills
Vicki Cline
W.K.

Bibliography

Allenowitz, Ralph, and Barbara Allenowitz. 2004. *Intimacy with impotence: A couples guide to better sex after prostate disease*. Boston: Da Capo Press.
Alves, Rubem. 1971. *A theology of hope*. Washington, DC: Corpus Books.
American Medical Association. 1977. First code of medical ethics. In *Ethics in medicine: Historical perspectives and contemporary concerns*, ed. Stanley Reiser, Arthur Dyck, and William Curran. Cambridge: MIT Press.
Applebaum, Paul. 2007. Assessment of patient's competency to consent to treatment. *New England Journal of Medicine* 351: 1834–1840.
Augustine. 1977. *The city of god*. Trans. Henry Bettenson. London: Penguin.
———. 1996. *Enchiridion: On faith, hope, and love*. Trans. Thomas Hibbs. Washington, DC: Regnery Publishing.
Bain, L.A. 1969. Marcels logic of freedom in proving the existence of god. *International Philosophical Quarterly* 9: 177–204.
Baker, R., Porter Dorthy, and Roger Porter. 1992. *The codification morality: Historical and philosophical studies in the formation of Western medical ethics*. New York: Springer.
Bakwin, Kanda, and Paul Komba. 2018. *Female genital mutilation*. New York: Springer.
Bedau, Hugo Adam, ed. 1997. *The death penalty in America*. London: Oxford University Press.
Benson, K. 1995. Refusal of transfusions by Jehovah's witnesses. *Cancer Control Journal* 2: 178–183.
Berg, J., et al. 1996. Constructing: Formulating standards of legal competence to make medical decisions. *Rutgers Law Review* 48: 345–396.
Billman, Brian, Patricia Lambert, and Banks Leonard. 2000. Cannibalism, warfare and drought in the Mesa Verde region during the twelfth century A.D. *American Antiquity* 65: 145–178.
Blechmann, M. 2008. Not yet: Adorno and the utopia of consciousness. *Cultural Critique* 70: 177–198.
Bloch, Ernst. 1921. *Thomas Munzer als Theologin der Revolution*. München: Wolff.
———. 1986. *The principle of hope*, 3 vols. Trans. Neville Place, Stephen Place, Paul Knight. Cambridge: MIT Press
———. 1988. *The utopian function of art and literature*. Eds. and Trans. Jack Zippes and Frank Mechlenberg. Cambridge.: MIT Press.
Blum, L. 1980. *Friendship, altruism and morality*. New York: Routledge.
Boldyrev, Ivan. 2014. *Ernst Bloch and his contemporaries: Locating utopian Messianism*. London: Bloomsbury Academic Publishers.
Bonner, Stuart. 2002. *The death Penalty: An American history*. Cambridge: Harvard University Press.

Braatan, Carl. 1969. *The future of god: The revolutionary dynamics of hope*. New York: Harper and Row.
Brang, D., et al. 2008. Aptomenophilia a neurological disorder. *Cognitive Neuroscience and Neuropsychology* 19: 1305–1306.
Brow, Peter. 2000. *Augustine of hippo: A biography*. 2nd ed. Berkeley: University of California Press.
Brown, R. 1988. *Analysing love*. London: Cambridge University Press.
Cabot, Richard Clarke. 1903. The uses of truth and falsehood in medicine. *American Medicine* 5: 344–349.
———. 1914. *Social science and the art of healing*. New York: Moffitt and Company.
———. 1919. *Social work: Essays on the meeting ground of doctor and social worker*. Boston: Houghton Mifflin.
———. 1931. What is worthwhile in nursing. *The American Journal of Nursing* 31: 277–285.
———. 1938. *Honesty*. New York: Macmillan Publishers.
Cabot, Richard Clarke, and Russel L. Dicks. 1936. *The art of ministering to the sick*. New York: Macmillan Publishers.
Calhoun, Cheshire. 2020. *Doing valuable time: The present, the future, and meaningful living*. London: Oxford University Press.
Callahan, Laura, and Timothy O'Connor. 2014. *Religious faith and intellectual virtue*. London: Oxford University Press.
Camus, Albert. 1948. *The plague*. Trans. Stuart Gilbert. New York: Random House.
Cappon, Donald. 1952. Attitudes of and toward the dying. *Canadian Medical Association Journal* 29: 693–700.
Castle, Lana. 2007. *Bipolar disorder demystified*. Boston: Da Capo Press.
Cohn, Norman. 1970. *The pursuit of the millennium: Revolutionary millenarians and mystical anarchists of the middle ages*. London: Oxford University Press.
Collins, Joseph. 1927. Should doctors tell the truth? *Harpers Monthly Magazine* 155: 320–326.
Day, J.P. 1967. Hope. *American Philosophical Quarterly* 6: 89–101.
De Garis, Hugo. 2006. *The Artilect Wars*. New York: ETC Publishing.
De Grazia, David. 2007. *Animal rights: A very short introduction*. London: Oxford University Press.
De Lisser, H.M., et al. 2009. The air got to it: Exploring a belief about surgery for lung cancer. *Journal of the National Medical Association* 10: 765–771.
Descartes, Rene. 1985. The passions of the soul. In *Philosophical writings of Descartes*, vol. 1. Eds. and Trans. John Cottingham, R. Southoff, D. Murdoch. London: Cambridge University Press.
Devita, D., and E. Chu. 2008. History of cancer chemotherapy. *Cancer Research* 68: 8643–8653.
Downie, Robin. 1963. Hope. *Philosophy and Phenomenological Research* 24: 248–251.
Easson, Eric. 1967. Cancer and the problem of pessimism. *CA—Cancer* 17: 7–14.
Elder, Lee. 2000. Why some Jehovah's witnesses accept blood and reject official blood policy. *Journal of Medical Ethics* 26: 375–380.
Elliot, Carl. 2000. A new way to be mad. *Atlantic Monthly* 286 (December): 72–84.
Engels, Friedrich. *Herr Eugen Duhring's revolution science:* Online at www.marxists.org.
Engels, Friedrich. *Socialism: Utopian and scientific*. Online at www.marxists.org.
Engels, Friedrich. *Speech at Marx's gravesite*. Online at www.marxists.org.
Fernandez, M.E., et al. 2008. Colorectal cancer screening among Latinos along the Texas–Mexico border. *Cancer Causes and Control* 19: 195–2006.
Findley, L.J., and P.M. Redstone. 1982. Blood transfusions in adult Jehovah's witnesses. *Archives of Internal Medicine* 142: 606–607.
First, M.B. 2005. Desire for amputation of a limb: Paraphilia, psychosis, or a new type of identity disorder. *Psychological Medicine* 35: 918–928.
Fitts, William, and I.S. Bowden. 1953. What Philadelphia physicians tell cancer patients. *Journal of the American Medical Association* 153: 901–904.
Fletcher, Joseph. 1974. *The ethics of genetic control*. New York: Anchor Books.
Fulton, Linda. 2016. *Hope: A comprehensive guide to living with and defeating manic depression*. Scotts Valley: Create Space Publishing.

Furth, G., and R. Smith. 2000. *Aptomenophilia: Information, questions, answers, and recommendations*. Bloomington: 1st Books Library.
Gay, Peter. 1952. *The dilemma of democratic socialism*. New York: Columbia University Press.
Geoghegan, Vincent. 1996. *Ernst Bloch*. New York: Routledge.
George, M., and M.R. Margolis. 2010. Race and lung cancer surgery: A qualitative analysis of relevant beliefs. *Oncology Nursing Forum* 37: 740–748.
Godfrey, J.J. 1987a. *A philosophy of human hope*. Dordrecht: Martinus Nijhoff.
———. 1987b. Appraising Marcel on hope. *Philosophy Today* 31: 234–240.
Gregg, J., and R.M. Curry. 1994. Explanatory models for cancer among African Americans at two Atlanta neighborhood hospitals: Implications for a health screening program. *Social Science and Medicine* 39: 519–526.
Gregory, John. 1772. *Duties and qualifications of a physician*. London: Strahan and Cadell.
Grisso, T., and Paul Applebaum. 1998. *Assessing competency to consent to medical care*. London: Oxford University Press.
Grossman, Terry, and Ray Kurzweil. 2005. *Fantastic voyage: How to live long enough to live forever*. New York: Plume.
Haakamsson, Lisbeth. 1997. *Medicine, and morals in the enlightenment*. Amsterdam: Rodophji Publishers.
Hanley, K.R., ed. 1998. *Gabriel Marcel's perspectives on a broken world*. Milwaukee: Marquette University Press.
Hartman, K., and Brian Long. 1999. Exceptions to informed consent in emergency medicine. *Hospital Medicine* 35: 53–55.
Haynes, Harley, and Richard Miles. 2021. *The prostate cancer owner's manual: What you need to know about diagnosis, treatment, and survival*. Baltimore: Rowman and Littlefield Publishers.
Helm, Paul. 2000. *Faith with knowledge*. London: Oxford University Press.
Helm, B. 2010. *Love, friendship, and the self*. London: Oxford University Press.
Hemming, John. 1979. *The search for El-Dorado*. New York: E.P. Dutton.
Hernandez, Jill. 2011. *Gabriel Marcel's ethics of Hope*. London: Bloomsbury Academic.
Herzog, Fredrick. 1972. *A theology of liberation*. New York: Seabury Press.
Hetrick, Jay. 2021. The uses and abuses of Bergson in critical theory. *Cosmos: The Journal of Natural and Social Philosophy* 17: 99–136.
Hick, John. 1966. *Faith and knowledge*. Ithaca: Cornell University Press.
Hobbes, Thomas. 1996. In *Leviathan*, ed. Richard Tuck. London: Cambridge University Press.
Holmes, Oliver Wendell. 1891. *Medical essays: 1842–1882*. Boston: Houghton Mifflin.
Horne, Alaister. 2012. *The fall of Paris: The Seige and the commune*. London: Picador Publishers.
Hudson, Wayne. 1982. *The Marxist philosophy of Ernst Bloch*. New York: St. Martin's Press.
James, William. 1982. *The verities of religious experience*. New York: Penguin Library.
Jameson, Kay Redfield. 1996. *An unquiet mind: A memoir of moods and madness*. New York: Vintage Publishers.
Jung, W. 1988. The early aesthetics of Bloch and Lukacs. *New German Critique* 45: 41–54.
Kadarsky, Arpad. 1991. *Georg Luckas: Life, thought, and politics*. London: Basil Blackwell Publishers.
Kalyvas, J., and N. Theodore. 2004. Lumbar spine stabilization. In *Encyclopedia of the neurological sciences*, ed. Michael Ominoff and Robert Doroff. Amsterdam: Elsevier Publishers.
Karadi, E. 1986. Bloch et Lukacs dans le cercle de Weber. In *Reification et utopia: Ernst Bloch et Gyorgy Lukacs un Siecle Apres*, ed. P. Furlan, M. Lowy, A. Munster, and N. Tertulian, 69–87. Arles: Actes Sud.
Kenny, Anthony. 1992. *What is faith?* London: Oxford University Press.
Kirshblum, Stephen, and Vernon Lin. 2018. *Spinal cord medicine*. 3rd ed. Cham: Demas Medical.
Kroeger, Katherine, et al. 2014. Effects of psychotherapy on patients suffering from body integrity disorder. *American Journal of Applied Psychotherapy* 3: 111–115.
Kubler-Ross, Elizabeth. 1969. *On death and dying*. New York: Macmillan Publishers.

Lambert, Patricia, Brian Billman, and Banks Leonard. 2000. Explaining variability in mutilated human bone assemblages in the southwest: A case study from the southern Piedmont of Sleeping Ute Mountain Colorado. *International Journal of Osteoarchaeology* 10: 49–64.

Langer, William. 1971. *The revolutions of 1848*. New York: Harper and Row Publishers.

Lanin, D.L., et al. 2002. Impacting cultural attitudes in African American women to decrease breast cancer morbidity. *American Journal of Surgery* 184: 918–922.

Leichtheim, George. 1964. *Marxism: A historical and critical study*. New York: Praeger Publishers.

Lewis, C.S. 2007. *The four loves*. New York: Harper and Row Publishers.

Lillenfeld, R. 1987. Music society in the 20th century: Georg Lukacs, Ernst Bloch, and Theodore Adorno. *International Journal of Politics, Culture, and Society* 1: 20–46.

Luft, Sebastian, ed. 2015. *The neo-Kantians*. New York: Routledge Publishers.

Mandary, Evan. 2011. *The death penalty in America*. Burlington: Jones and Bartlett.

Margolis, M.L., et al. 2003. Racial differences pertaining to beliefs about lung cancer surgery. *Annals of Internal Medicine* 139: 558–562.

Marson, D., et al. 1995. Assessing the competency of patients with Alzheimer's disease under different legal standards. *Archives of Neurology* 52: 949–959.

Masi, C.M., and S. Gehlert. 2008. Perceptions of breast cancer surgery among African American women and men. *Journal of General Medicine* 24: 408–414.

McCown, Joe. 1978. *Availability: Gabriel Marcel and the phenomenology of human openness*. Missoula: Scholars Press.

McGoech, P.D., et al. 2009. Apotemnophilia: The neurological basis of a psychological disorder. *Nature Proceedings* 4: 1–5.

Meeks, Douglas. 1974. *Origins of the theology of hope*. Philadelphia: Fortress Press.

Meirav, Ariel. 2008. The nature of hope. *Ratio* 22: 216–233.

Mendes-Flohr, P. 1983. To brush history against the grain: The eschatology of the Frankfurt School and Ernst Bloch. *Journal of the American Academy of Religion* 51: 631–649.

Michaelson, Brittany. 2020. *Voices for animal liberation*. New York: Skyhorse Press.

Moltmonn, Jurgen. 1965. *The theology of hope: On the grounding and implications of Christian eschatology*. Trans. James Leitch. London: S.C.M. Press.

Moore, Adrienne, ed. 2018. *The Routledge handbook of love in philosophy*. New York: Routledge.

Mulhall, John. 2008. *Saving your sex life: A guide for men with prostate cancer*. Chicago: Hilton Publishers.

Murdoch, Jessica. 2014. Between heaven and history: Rahner on hope. *New Blackfriers* 95: 263–284.

Neff, D., and E. Kasten. 2010. Body identity integrity disorder: What do health professionals know? *European Journal of Counselling Psychology* 1: 16–30.

Nussbaum, Martha. 1999. *Sex and social justice*. London: Oxford University Press.

O'Brien, T.C. 1974. *Faith in St. Thomas Aquinas*. London: Basil Blackwell.

Oaken, Donald. 1961. What to tell cancer patients? *Journal of the American Medical Association* 175: 1120–1128.

Pannenberg, Wolfhart. 1969. *Theology and the kingdom of god*. Trans. Richard John Neuhaus. Philadelphia: Westminster Press.

Pearson, Angell. 2011. *Henri Bergson: An introduction*. New York: Routledge.

Penelhum, Terence, ed. 1989. *Faith*. London: Collier Macmillan.

Percival, Thomas. 1803. *Medical ethics: A code of institutes and precepts adapted to the professional interests of physicians and surgeons*. Manchester: S. Russel and Co.

Pettit, Phillip. 2004. Hope and its place in mind. *Annals of the American Academy of Political and Social Science* 592: 152–165.

Rabinbach, A. 1997. *In the shadow of catastrophe: German intellectuals between apocalypse and enlightenment*. Berkley: University of California Press.

Radnoti, S. 1975. Bloch and Lukacs: Two radical critics in a god forsaken world. *Telos* 25: 156–166.

Randall, A. 1992. *The mystery of hope in the philosophy of Gabriel Marcel*. New York: Mellen Press.

Regan, Tom. 2004. *The case for animal rights*. Berkeley: University of California Press.

Richard, Sherlock, and C. Mary Dingus. 1985. Families and the gravely ill: Roles, rules, and rights. *Journal of the American Geriatric Society* 33: 121–124.

Richter, G. 2006. Bloch's dreams: Music's traces. In *Sound figures of modernity: German music and philosophy*, ed. J. Hermand and G. Richter, 141–180. Madison: University of Wisconsin Press.

Roberts, Richard. 1990. *Hope and heiroglyphs: A critical decipherment of Ernst Bloch's "principle of hope"*. Atlanta: Scholars Press.

Sarischoulis, Efstraios. 2016. Fate, free will and narrative in Homeric epics. *Mythos* 10: 81–115.

Scott, Tom. 1989. *Thomas Muntzer: Theology and revolution in the German reformation*. London: Macmillan Publishers.

Segal, M.G. 1943. Should cancer victims be told the truth? *Missouri Medical Association* 40: 33–35.

Segal, Andrew. 2019. *Prostate cancer 2020: A practical guide to understanding, management, and treatment options for patients and their families*. Louisville: Rogue Wave Press.

Sessions, William. 1994. *The concept of faith*. Ithaca: Cornell University Press.

Shaffer, Peter. 1975. *Equus*. New York: Avon Books.

Singer, I. 1984–1989. *Tshe nature of love*, 3 vols. Chicago: University of Chicago Press.

Skaine, Rosemary. 2005. *Female genital mutilation: Legal, cultural, and medical issues*. Jefferson: McFarland Publishers.

Smith, Cameron, and Evan Davis. 2012. *Emigrating beyond earth*. New York: Springer.

Soble, A. 1989. *Eros, agape, and friendship: Readings in the philosophy of love*. New York: Paragon Press.

Steeger, Manfred. 1997. *The quest for evolutionary socialism*. London: Cambridge University Press.

Steenson, Gary. 1978. *Karl Kautsky: 1885–1938, Marxism in the classical years*. Pittsburgh: University of Pittsburgh Press.

Steerns, Peter. 2005. *The revolutionary tide in Europe*. London: Oxford University Press.

Styap, Jules. 1870. *A code of medical ethics*. London: Churchill Publishers.

Sweetman, Brendan. 2008. *The vision of Gabriel Marcel: Epistemology, human person, the transcendent*. Amsterdam: Rodopi Press.

———, ed. 2011. *A Gabriel Marcel reader*. South Bend: St. Augustine's Press.

Teresa of Avila. 1997. *The life of St. Teresa of Avila*. Ed. Benedict Zimmerman. Trans. David Lewis. Gastonia: Tan Books.

Thompson, P. 2013. *The privatization of hope: Ernst Bloch and the future of utopia*. Durham: Duke University Press.

Tombs, Robert. 2014. *The Paris commune*. New York: Routledge.

Torrey, E. Fuller, and Michael Knoble. 2005. *Surviving manic depression*. New York: Basic Books.

Verdwaerdt, Adrian, and Debbie Wilson. 1967. Communicating with terminally ill patients. *American Journal of Nursing* 67: 230–239.

Vidal-Naguet, Pierre. 2007. *The Atlantis story: A short history of Plato's myth*. Exeter: Exeter University Press.

Virgil. 1985. *The Aeneid*. Trans. Robert Fitzgerald. New York: Random House Publishers.

Von Hildebrandt, Dietrich. 2010. *The nature of love*. Trans. John Crosby. Notre Dame: St. Augustine Press.

Waddi Ton, Ivan. 1975. The development of medical ethics. *Medical History* 19: 38–51ng.

Wear, Andrew, and Johann Kordesch, eds. 1993. *Doctors and ethics: The earlier selling of professional ethics*. Amsterdam: Rodopi.

Weissberg, L. 1992. Philosophy and fairy tales: Ernst Bloch as narrator. *New German Criticism* 55: 21–44.

Weitzel, James. 2012. *Augustine's city of god: A critical guide*. London: Cambridge University Press.

West, Thomas. 1991. *Ultimate hope without god: The atheist eschatology of Ernst Bloch*. New York: Peter Lang.

Whalen, Bernard. 2009. *The dominion of god: Christianity and apocalypse in the Middle Ages*. Cambridge: Harvard University Press.

Wood, Charles. 1946. The doctor, the patient, and the truth. *Annals of Internal Medicine* 24: 955–959.

Author Index

A
Abraham, 62, 63, 74
Al Khutwa, 58
Al Shah, 58
Armstrong, N., 71, 84

B
Babel, A., 64
Bergson, H., 67, 68
Bernstein, E., 64
Bloch, E., 4, 65–73, 75

C
Calhoun, C., 51
Castel, 26–28, 32, 33, 57, 58, 83
Collins, J., 9, 11
Cook, J., 84

D
Davis, M., 22, 29
Day, J.P., 51, 52, 55
Descartes, R., 52
Downie, R., 51, 52, 54, 55, 59
Dysart, M., 41–44, 58, 82, 84

E
Engles, F., 64, 65

F
Flandro, P., 25, 26, 31, 32, 79

G
Gupta, 24, 30, 33, 35, 53, 89

H
Henkson, G., 22, 23, 29, 30, 52, 89
Hildegard of Bingen, 58, 65
Hitler, 55, 57, 66
Hobbes, T., 52
Holmes, O.W., 7–12, 47

I
Ibn Arabi, 58

J
Joachim of Fiore, 66, 69
John of the Cross, 44, 58

K
Kautsky, K., 64–66
Kubler-Ross, E., 11, 12, 47, 54

L
Lukacs, G., 65, 68

M
Marcel, G., 76, 77, 79–82, 85–88, 91
Martin, L., 25
Marx, K., 63–66, 72, 73
Meirav, A., 54
Miller, J., 23, 24
Moses, 10, 63, 72, 90
Muntzer, T., 66

O
Oaken, D., 10, 11
Othon, M., 28, 32

P
Paneloux, Fr., 26, 28, 58
Percival, T., 1–3, 5–17, 27, 47, 58, 89, 91
Pettit, P., 51

R
Rieux, B., 26–29, 32, 33, 35, 57, 58, 83

S
Steel, K., 24, 30, 33, 84, 88, 89
Strang, A., 58, 82, 84
Strang, D., 41

T
Teresa of Avila, 42, 43, 58

W
Williams, D., 39, 46
Wilson, L., 25, 31

Subject Index

A
Absolute Thou, 88
American College of Physicians, 16
American Medical Association Code 1849, 1, 6
American Medical Association Principles 1903, 8
Aptomenophilia, 36, 37

B
Biopsy, 20, 46
Blueprint Marxism, 68
Broken world, 77, 78, 80, 84, 87–89, 91

C
Capital punishment, 56
Celexa, 23
Christ, 14, 41–43, 50, 72
Christianity, 4, 8, 54, 66, 72
City of God, 61, 62, 67, 75
Clonazepam, 22
Competency, 38, 46
Confidentiality, 1, 32
Crohn's disease, 37
CT scans, 23, 25

D
Darkness, 28, 46, 80, 87
Depakote, 22, 23
Depression, 22, 23, 29, 30, 36, 45
Disordered hope, 57

E
Equus, 41–43, 82, 83
External factor, 54

F
Faiths, 2, 4, 5, 12, 14, 28, 30, 40–45, 50, 67, 76–78, 80, 82–92
Fantastic Voyage, 53
Female circumcision, 56

H
Holy Spirit, 43, 44, 47, 66
Hope and desire, 65, 74
Hope and uncertainty, 51–54
Hungarian American, 81

I
Inform the family, 7, 24
Institute for Social Research, 66

J
Jehovah's Witnesses, 40, 45

K
Kabbala, 58

L
Lithium, 23
Love, 4–6, 10, 15, 22, 30, 40, 42, 49, 50, 61, 80

M
Manic depression, 22, 23, 29, 70, 73, 89
Marxism, 63–66, 69, 73
Medical social work, 13
Minister of hope, 2, 4, 6, 8, 47, 89, 91
Miracles, 3, 12, 30, 58, 84
Moral relativism, 56
Mormons, 62, 75
Mythic figures, 72

N
Narcotic analgesics, 25
Nasogastric tube, 37, 39, 46
New York Giants, 51

O
Optimism, 4, 9, 32, 69, 86
Orthopedic surgeons, 36, 78

P
Paris Commune, 64
Paxil, 22, 29
Problem and mystery, 77–82
Promised land, 62
Prostate cancer, 21, 30, 31, 78
Psychology of Hope, 4
Puritans, 62

R
Referential thinking, 22
Religions, 2, 4, 6, 8, 13, 15, 41, 42, 44, 53–55, 67, 72, 73, 81

S
Schizophrenia, 39, 46, 70
Self-amputation, 37, 41
Seroquel, 22, 23
Sexual intimacy, 21, 29, 31, 32
Spinal column, 22, 25, 75

T
Temporal goods, 3, 61–63, 73–74, 86
Teresa of Avila, 42, 43, 58
Theology of Hope, 4, 67
The plague, 24, 26–28, 57, 83
Truth to the patient, 8–11, 16

U
Unitarians, 14
Urinary continence, 21, 25, 32, 78

Z
Zohar, 58

SPRINGER NATURE

GPSR Compliance

The European Union's (EU) General Product Safety Regulation (GPSR) is a set of rules that requires consumer products to be safe and our obligations to ensure this.

If you have any concerns about our products, you can contact us on ProductSafety@springernature.com

In case Publisher is established outside the EU, the EU authorized representative is:

Springer Nature Customer Service Center GmbH
Europaplatz 3
69115 Heidelberg, Germany

The manufacturer's authorised representative in the EU is Springer Nature Customer Service Centre GmbH, Europaplatz 3, 69115 Heidelberg, Germany. If you have any concerns regarding our products, please contact ProductSafety@springernature.com

Printed and bound by CPI Group (UK) Ltd, Croydon, CR0 4YY

26/03/2026

02078916-0010